THE ELEP
AND OTHER R

To secure Merrick's recovery and to bring him, as it were, to life once more, it was necessary that he should make the acquaintance of men and women who would treat him as a normal and intelligent young man and not as a monster of deformity.

I asked a friend of mine, a young and pretty widow, if she thought she could enter Merrick's room with a smile, wish him good morning and shake him by the hand. She said she could and she did. The effect upon poor Merrick was not quite what I had expected. As he let go her hand he bent his head on his knees and sobbed until I thought he would never cease. The interview was over. He told me afterwards that this was the first woman who had ever smiled at him, and the first woman, in the whole of his life, who had shaken hands with him.

THE ELEPHANT MAN
AND OTHER REMINISCENCES

Sir Frederick Treves

A STAR BOOK

published by
the Paperback Division of
W. H. ALLEN & Co. Ltd

A Star Book
Published in 1980
by the Paperback Division of
W. H. Allen & Co. Ltd
A Howard and Wyndham Company
44 Hill Street, London W1X 8LB

First published in Great Britain by
Cassell & Co., 1923

Printed in Great Britain by
C. Nicholls & Company Ltd, The Philips Park Press, Manchester

ISBN 0 352 307471

CONTENTS

THE ELEPHANT MAN

In the Mile End Road, opposite to the London Hospital, there was (and possibly still is) a line of small shops. Among them was a vacant greengrocer's which was to let. The whole of the front of the shop, with the exception of the door, was hidden by a hanging sheet of canvas on which was the announcement that the Elephant Man was to be seen within and that the price of admission was twopence. Painted on the canvas in primitive colours was a life-size portrait of the Elephant Man. This very crude production depicted a frightful creature that could only have been possible in a nightmare. It was the figure of a man with the characteristics of an elephant. The transfiguration was not far advanced. There was still more of the man than of the beast. This fact – that it was still human – was the most repellent attribute of the creature. There was nothing about it of the pitiableness of the misshapened or the deformed, nothing of the grotesqueness of the freak, but merely the loathsome insinuation of a man being changed into an animal. Some palm trees in the background of the picture suggested a jungle and might have led the imaginative to assume that it was in this wild that the perverted object had roamed.

When I first became aware of this phenomenon the exhibition was closed, but a well-informed boy sought the proprietor in a public house and I was granted a private view on payment of a shilling. The shop was empty and grey with dust. Some old tins and a few shrivelled potatoes occupied a shelf and some vague vegetable refuse the window. The light in the place was dim, being obscured by the painted placard outside. The far end of the shop – where I expect the late proprietor sat at a desk – was cut off by a curtain or rather by a red tablecloth suspended from a cord by a few rings. The room was cold and dank, for it was the month of November. The year, I might say, was 1884.

The showman pulled back the curtain and revealed a bent figure crouching on a stool and covered by a brown blanket. In front of it, on a tripod, was a large brick heated by a Bunsen burner. Over this the creature was huddled to warm itself. It never moved when the curtain was drawn back. Locked up in an empty shop and lit by the faint blue light of the gas jet, this hunched-up figure was the embodiment of loneliness. It might have been a captive in a cavern or a wizard watching for unholy manifestations in the ghostly flame. Outside the sun was shining and one could hear the footsteps of the passers-by, a tune whistled by a boy and the companionable hum of traffic in the road.

The showman – speaking as if to a dog – called out harshly: 'Stand up!' The thing arose slowly and let the blanket that covered its head and back fall to the ground. There stood revealed the most disgusting specimen of humanity that I have ever seen. In the course of my profession I had come upon lamentable deformities of the face due to injury or disease, as well as mutilations and contortions of the body depending upon like causes; but at no time had I met with such a degraded or perverted version of a human being as this lone figure displayed. He was naked to the waist, his feet were bare, he wore a pair of threadbare trousers that had once belonged to some fat gentleman's dress suit.

From the intensified painting in the street I had imagined the Elephant Man to be of gigantic size. This, however, was a little man below the average height and made to look shorter by the bowing of his back. The most striking feature about him was his enormous and misshapened head. From the brow there projected a huge bony mass like a loaf, while from the back of the head hung a bag of spongy, fungous-looking skin, the surface of which was comparable to brown cauli-flower. On the top of the skull were a few long lank hairs. The osseous growth on the forehead almost occluded one eye. The circumference of the head was no less than that of the man's waist. From the upper jaw there projected another mass of bone. It protruded from the mouth like a pink stump, turning the upper lip inside out and making of the mouth a mere slobbering aperture. This growth from the jaw had been so exaggerated in the painting as to appear to be a rudimentary trunk or tusk. The nose was merely a lump of flesh, only recognizable as a nose from its position. The face was no more capable of expression than a block of gnarled wood. The back was horrible, because from it hung, as far down as the middle of the thigh, huge, sack-like masses of flesh covered by the same loathsome cauliflower skin.

The right arm was of enormous size and shapeless. It suggested the limb of the subject of elephantiasis. It was overgrown also with pendent masses of the same cauliflower-like skin. The hand was large and clumsy – a fin or paddle rather than a hand. There was no distinction between the palm and the back. The thumb had the appearance of a radish, while the fingers might have been thick, tuberous roots. As a limb it was almost useless. The other arm was remarkable by contrast. It was not only normal but was, moreover, a delicately shaped limb covered with fine skin and provided with a beautiful hand which any woman might have envied. From the chest hung a bag of the same repulsive flesh. It was like a dewlap suspended from the neck of a lizard. The lower limbs had the characters of the deformed arm. They were unwieldy, dropsical looking and grossly misshapened.

To add a further burden to his trouble the wretched man, when a boy, developed hip disease, which had left him permanently lame, so that he could only walk with a stick. He was thus denied all means of escape from his tormentors. As he told me later, he could never run away. One other feature must be mentioned to emphasize his isolation from his kind. Although he was already repellent enough, there arose from the fungous skin-growth with which he was almost covered a very sickening stench which was hard to tolerate. From the showman I learnt nothing about the Elephant Man, except that he was English, that his name was John Merrick and that he was twenty-one years of age.

As at the time of my discovery of the Elephant Man I was the Lecturer on Anatomy at the Medical College opposite, I was anxious to examine him in detail and to prepare an account of his abnormalities. I therefore arranged with the showman that I should interview his strange exhibit in my room at the college. I became at once conscious of a difficulty. The Elephant Man could not show himself in the streets. He would have been mobbed by the crowd and seized by the police. He was, in fact, as secluded from the world as the Man with the Iron Mask. He had, however, a disguise, although it was almost as startling as he was himself. It consisted of a long black cloak which reached to the ground. Whence the cloak had been obtained I cannot imagine. I had only seen such a garment on the stage wrapped about the figure of a Venetian bravo. The recluse was provided with a pair of bag-like slippers in which to hide his deformed feet. On his head was a cap of a kind that never before was seen. It was black like the cloak, had a wide peak, and the general outline of a yachting cap. As the circumference of Merrick's head was that of a man's waist, the size of this headgear may be imagined. From the attachment of the peak a grey flannel curtain hung in front of the face. In this mask was cut a wide horizontal slit through which the wearer could look out. This costume, worn by a bent man hobbling along with a stick, is probably the most remarkable and the most uncanny that has as yet been designed. I arranged that Merrick should cross the road in a cab, and to insure his immediate admission to the college I gave him my card. This card was destined to play a critical part in Merrick's life.

I made a careful examination of my visitor the result of which I embodied in a paper.* I made little of the man himself. He was shy, confused, not a little frightened and evidently much cowed. Moreover, his speech was almost unintelligible. The great bony mass that projected from his mouth blurred his utterance and made the articulation of certain words impossible. He returned in a cab to the place of exhibition, and I assumed that I had seen the last of him,

*British Medical Journal, Dec., 1886, and April, 1890.

especially as I found next day that the show had been forbidden by the police and that the shop was empty.

I supposed that Merrick was imbecile and had been imbecile from birth. The fact that his face was incapable of expression, that his speech was a mere spluttering and his attitude that of one whose mind was void of all emotions and concerns gave grounds for this belief. The conviction was no doubt encouraged by the hope that his intellect was the blank I imagined it to be. That he could appreciate his position was unthinkable. Here was a man in the heyday of youth who was so vilely deformed that everyone he met confronted him with a look of horror and disgust. He was taken about the country to be exhibited as a monstrosity and an object of loathing. He was shunned like a leper, housed like a wild beast, and got his only view of the world from a peephole in a showman's cart. He was, moreover, lame, had but one available arm, and could hardly make his utterances understood. It was not until I came to know that Merrick was highly intelligent, that he possessed an acute sensibility and – worse than all – a romantic imagination that I realized the overwhelming tragedy of his life.

The episode of the Elephant Man was, I imagined, closed; but I was fated to meet him again – two years later – under more dramatic conditions. In England the showman and Merrick had been moved on from place to place by the police, who considered the exhibition degrading and among the things that could not be allowed. It was hoped that in the uncritical retreats of Mile End a more abiding peace would be found. But it was not to be. The official mind there, as elsewhere, very properly decreed that the public exposure of Merrick and his deformities transgressed the limits of decency. The show must close.

The showman, in despair, fled with his charge to the Continent. Whither he roamed at first I do not know; but he came finally to Brussels. His reception was discouraging. Brussels was firm; the exhibition was banned; it was brutal, indecent and immoral, and could not be permitted within the confines of Belgium. Merrick was thus no longer of value. He

11

was no longer a source of profitable entertainment. He was a burden. He must be got rid of. The elimination of Merrick was a simple matter. He could offer no resistance. He was as docile as a sick sheep. The impresario, having robbed Merrick of his paltry savings, gave him a ticket to London, saw him into the train and no doubt in parting condemned him to perdition.

His destination was Liverpool Street. The journey may be imagined. Merrick was in his alarming outdoor garb. He would be harried by an eager mob as he hobbled along the quay. They would run ahead to get a look at him. They would lift the hem of his cloak to peep at his body. He would try to hide in the train or in some dark corner of the boat, but never could he be free from that ring of curious eyes or from those whispers of fright and aversion. He had but a few shillings in his pocket and nothing either to eat or drink on the way. A panic-dazed dog with a label on his collar would have received some sympathy and possibly some kindness. Merrick received none.

What was he to do when he reached London? He had not a friend in the world. He knew no more of London than he knew of Pekin. How could he find a lodging, or what lodging-house keeper would dream of taking him in? All he wanted was to hide. What most he dreaded were the open street and the gaze of his fellow-men. If even he crept into a cellar the horrid eyes and the still more dreaded whispers would follow him to its depths. Was there ever such a homecoming!

At Liverpool Street he was rescued from the crowd by the police and taken into the third-class waiting-room. Here he sank on the floor in the darkest corner. The police were at a loss what to do with him. They had dealt with strange and mouldy tramps, but never with such an object as this. He could not explain himself. His speech was so maimed that he might as well have spoken in Arabic. He had, however, something with him which he produced with a ray of hope. It was my card.

The card simplified matters. It made it evident that this

12

curious creature had an acquaintance and that the individual must be sent for. A messenger was dispatched to the London Hospital which is comparatively near at hand. Fortunately I was in the building and returned at once with the messenger to the station. In the waiting-room I had some difficulty in making a way through the crowd, but there, on the floor in the corner, was Merrick. He looked a mere heap. It seemed as if he had been thrown there like a bundle. He was so huddled up and so helpless looking that he might have had both his arms and his legs broken. He seemed pleased to see me, but he was nearly done. The journey and want of food had reduced him to the last stage of exhaustion. The police kindly helped him into a cab, and I drove him at once to the hospital. He appeared to be content, for he fell asleep almost as soon as he was seated and slept to the journey's end. He never said a word, but seemed to be satisfied that all was well.

In the attics of the hospital was an isolation ward with a single bed. It was used for emergency purposes – for a case of delirium tremens, for a man who had become suddenly insane or for a patient with an undetermined fever. Here the Elephant Man was deposited on a bed, was made comfortable and was supplied with food. I had been guilty of an irregularity in admitting such a case, for the hospital was neither a refuge nor a home for incurables. Chronic cases were not accepted, but only those requiring active treatment, and Merrick was not in need of such treatment. I applied to the sympathetic chairman of the committee, Mr. Carr Gomm, who not only was good enough to approve my action but who agreed with me that Merrick must not again be turned out into the world.

Mr. Carr Gomm wrote a letter to the *Times* detailing the circumstances of the refugee and asking for money for his support. So generous is the English public that in a few days – I think in a week – enough money was forthcoming to maintain Merrick for life without any charge upon the hospital funds. There chanced to be two empty rooms at the back of the hospital which were little used. They were on the ground floor, were out of the way, and opened upon a large courtyard called Bedstead Square, because here the iron beds were marshalled for cleaning and painting. The front room was converted into a bed-sitting room and the smaller chamber into a bathroom. The condition of Merrick's skin rendered a bath at least once a day a necessity, and I might here mention that with the use of the bath the unpleasant odour to which I have referred ceased to be noticeable. Merrick took up his abode in the hospital in December, 1886.

Merrick had now something he had never dreamed of, never supposed to be possible – a home of his own for life. I at once began to make myself acquainted with him and to endeavour to understand his mentality. It was a study of much interest. I very soon learnt his speech so that I could talk freely with him. This afforded him great satisfaction, for, curiously enough, he had a passion for conversation, yet all his life had had had no one to talk to. I – having then much leisure – saw him almost every day, and made a point of spending some two hours with him every Sunday morning when he would chatter almost without ceasing. It was unreasonable to expect one nurse to attend to him continuously, but there was no lack of temporary volunteers. As they did not all acquire his speech it came about that I had occasionally to act as an interpreter.

I found Merrick, as I have said, remarkably intelligent. He had learnt to read and had become a most voracious reader. I think he had been taught when he was in hospital with his diseased hip. His range of books was limited. The Bible and Prayer Book he knew intimately, but he had subsisted for the most part upon newspapers, or rather upon such fragments of old journals as he had chanced to pick up. He had read a few stories and some elementary lesson books, but the delight of his life was a romance, especially a love romance. These tales were very real to him, as real as any narrative in the Bible, so that he would tell them to me as incidents in the lives of people who had lived. In his outlook upon the world he was a child, yet a child with some of the tempestuous feelings of a man. He was an elemental being, so primitive

14

that he might have spent the twenty-three years of his life immured in a cave.

Of his early days I could learn but little. He was very loath to talk about the past. It was a nightmare, the shudder of which was still upon him. He was born, he believed, in or about Leicester. Of his father he knew absolutely nothing. Of his mother he had some memory. It was very faint and had, I think, been elaborated in his mind into something definite. Mothers figured in the tales he had read, and he wanted his mother to be one of those comfortable lullaby-singing persons who are so lovable. In his subconscious mind there was apparently a germ of recollection in which someone figured who had been kind to him. He clung to this conception and made it more real by invention, for since the day when he could toddle no one had been kind to him. As an infant he must have been repellent, although his deformities did not become gross until he had attained his full stature.

It was a favourite belief of his that his mother was beautiful. The fiction was, I am aware, one of his own making, but it was a great joy to him. His mother, lovely as she may have been, basely deserted him when he was very small, so small that his earliest clear memories were of the workhouse to which he had been taken. Worthless and inhuman as this mother was, he spoke of her with pride and even with reverence. Once, when referring to his own appearance, he said: 'It *is* very strange, for, you see, mother was so beautiful.'

The rest of Merrick's life up to the time that I met him at Liverpool Street Station was one dull record of degradation and squalor. He was dragged from town to town and from fair to fair as if he were a strange beast in a cage. A dozen times a day he would have to expose his nakedness and his piteous deformities before a gaping crowd who greeted him with such mutterings as 'Oh! What a horror! What a beast!' He had had no childhood. He had had no boyhood. He had never experienced pleasure. He knew nothing of the joy of living nor of the fun of things. His sole idea of happiness was to creep into the dark and hide. Shut up alone in a booth, awaiting the next exhibition, how mocking must have

15

sounded the laughter and merriment of the boys and girls outside who were enjoying the 'fun of the fair'! He had no past to look back upon and no future to look forward to. At the age of twenty he was a creature without hope. There was nothing in front of him but a vista of caravans creeping along a road, of rows of glaring show tents and of circles of staring eyes with, at the end, the spectacle of a broken man in a poor law infirmary.

Those who are interested in the evolution of character might speculate as to the effect of this brutish life upon a sensitive and intelligent man. It would be reasonable to surmise that he would become a spiteful and malignant misanthrope, swollen with venom and filled with hatred of his fellow-men, or, on the other hand, that he would degenerate into a despairing melancholic on the verge of idiocy. Merrick, however, was no such being. He had passed through the fire and had come out unscathed. His troubles had ennobled him. He showed himself to be a gentle, affectionate and lovable creature, as amiable as a happy woman, free from any trace of cynicism or resentment, without a grievance and without an unkind word for anyone. I have never heard him complain. I have never heard him deplore his ruined life or resent the treatment he had received at the hands of callous keepers. His journey through life had been indeed along a *via dolorosa*, the road had been uphill all the way, and now, when the night was at its blackest and the way most steep, he had suddenly found himself, as it were, in a friendly inn, bright with light and warm with welcome. His gratitude to those about him was pathetic in its sincerity and eloquent in the childlike simplicity with which it was expressed.

As I learnt more of this primitive creature I found that there were two anxieties which were prominent in his mind and which he revealed to me with diffidence. He was in the occupation of the rooms assigned to him and had been assured that he would be cared for to the end of his days. This, however, he found hard to realize, for he often asked me timidly to what place he would next be moved. To understand his attitude it is necessary to remember that he had been moving on and moving on all his life. He knew no other state of existence. To him it was normal. He had passed from the workhouse to the hospital, from the hospital back to the workhouse, then from this town to that town or from one showman's caravan to another. He had never known a home nor any semblance of one. He had no possessions. His sole belongings, besides his clothes and some books, were the monstrous cap and the cloak. He was a wanderer, a pariah and an outcast. That his quarters at the hospital were his for life he could not understand. He could not rid his mind of the anxiety which had pursued him for so many years – where am I to be taken next?

Another trouble was his dread of his fellow men, his fear of people's eyes, the dread of being always stared at, the lash of the cruel mutterings of the crowd. In his home in Bedstead Square he was secluded; but now and then a thoughtless porter or a wardmaid would open his door to let curious friends have a peep at the Elephant Man. It therefore seemed to him as if the gaze of the world followed him still.

Influenced by these two obsessions he became, during his first few weeks at the hospital, curiously uneasy. At last, with much hesitation, he said to me one day: 'When I am next moved can I go to a blind asylum or to a lighthouse?' He had read about blind asylums in the newspapers and was attracted by the thought of being among people who could not see. The lighthouse had another charm. It meant seclusion from the curious. There at least no one could open a door and peep in at him. There he would forget that he had once been the Elephant Man. There he would escape the vampire showman. He had never seen a lighthouse, but he had come upon a picture of the Eddystone, and it appeared to him that this lonely column of stone in the waste of the sea was such a home as he had longed for.

I had no great difficulty in ridding Merrick's mind of these ideas. I wanted him to get accustomed to his fellow-men, to become a human being himself and to be admitted to the communion of his kind. He appeared day by day less frightened, less haunted looking, less anxious to hide, less alarmed when he saw his door being opened. He got to know most of the people about the place, to be accustomed to their comings and goings, and to realize that they took no more than a friendly notice of him. He could only go out after dark, and on fine nights ventured to take a walk in Bedstead Square clad in his black cloak and his cap. His greatest adventure was on one moonless evening when he walked alone as far as the hospital garden and back again.

To secure Merrick's recovery and to bring him, as it were, to life once more, it was necessary that he should make the acquaintance of men and women who would treat him as a normal and intelligent young man and not as a monster of deformity. Women I felt to be more important than men in bringing about his transformation. Women were the more frightened of him, the more disgusted at his appearance and the more apt to give way to irrepressible expressions of aversion when they came into his presence. Moreover, Merrick had an admiration of women of such a kind that it attained almost to adoration. This was not the outcome of his personal experience. They were not real women but the products of his imagination. Among them was the beautiful mother surrounded, at a respectful distance, by heroines from the many romances he had read.

His first entry to the hospital was attended by a regrettable incident. He had been placed on the bed in the little attic, and a nurse had been instructed to bring him some food. Unfortunately she had not been fully informed of Merrick's unusual appearance. As she entered the room she saw on the bed, propped up by white pillows, a monstrous figure as hideous as an Indian idol. She at once dropped the tray she was carrying and fled, with a shriek, through the door. Merrick was too weak to notice much, but the experience, I am afraid, was not new to him.

He was looked after by volunteer nurses whose ministrations were somewhat formal and constrained. Merrick, no doubt, was conscious that their service was purely official, that they were merely doing what they were told to do and that they were acting rather as automata than as women.

They did not help him to feel that he was of their kind. On the contrary they, without knowing it, made him aware that the gulf of separation was immeasurable.

Feeling this, I asked a friend of mine, a young and pretty widow, if she thought she could enter Merrick's room with a smile, wish him good morning and shake him by the hand. She said she could and she did. The effect upon poor Merrick was not quite what I had expected. As he let go her hand he bent his head on his knees and sobbed until I thought he would never cease. The interview was over. He told me afterwards that this was the first woman who had ever smiled at him, and the first woman, in the whole of his life, who had shaken hands with him. From this day the transformation of Merrick commenced and he began to change, little by little, from a hunted thing into a man. It was a wonderful change to witness and one that never ceased to fascinate me.

Merrick's case attracted much attention in the papers, with the result that he had a constant succession of visitors. Everybody wanted to see him. He must have been visited by almost every lady of note in the social world. They were all good enough to welcome him with a smile and to shake hands with him. The Merrick whom I had found shivering behind a rag of a curtain in an empty shop was now conversant with duchesses and countesses and other ladies of high degree. They brought him presents, made his room bright with ornaments and pictures, and, what pleased him more than all, supplied him with books. He soon had a large library and most of his day was spent in reading. He was not the least spoiled; not the least puffed up; he never asked for anything; never presumed upon the kindness meted out to him, and was always humbly and profoundly grateful. Above all he lost his shyness. He liked to see his door pushed open and people to look in. He became acquainted with most of the frequenters of Bedstead Square, would chat with them at his window and show them some of his choicest presents. He improved in his speech, although to the end his utterances were not easy for strangers to understand. He was beginning, moreoever, to be less conscious of his unsightliness, a little

19

disposed to think it was, after all, not so very extreme. Possibly this was aided by the circumstance that I would not allow a mirror of any kind in his room.

The height of his social development was reached on an eventful day when Queen Alexandra – then Princess of Wales – came to the hospital to pay him a special visit. With that kindness which has marked every act of her life, the Queen entered Merrick's room smiling and shook him warmly by the hand. Merrick was transported with delight. This was beyond even his most extravagant dream. The Queen has made many people happy, but I think no gracious act of hers has ever caused such happiness as she brought into Merrick's room when she sat by his chair and talked to him as to a person she was glad to see.

Merrick, I may say, was now one of the most contented creatures I have chanced to meet. More than once he said to me: 'I am happy every hour of the day.' This was good to think upon when I recalled the half-dead heap of miserable humanity I had seen in the corner of the waiting-room at Liverpool Street. Most men of Merrick's age would have expressed their joy and sense of contentment by singing or whistling when they were alone. Unfortunately poor Merrick's mouth was so deformed that he could neither whistle nor sing. He was satisfied to express himself by beating time upon the pillow to some tune that was ringing in his head. I have many times found him so occupied when I have entered his room unexpectedly. One thing that always struck me as sad about Merrick was the fact that he could not smile. Whatever his delight might be, his face remained expressionless. He could weep but he could not smile.

The Queen paid Merrick many visits and sent him every year a Christmas card with a message in her own handwriting. On one occasion she sent him a signed photograph of herself. Merrick, quite overcome, regarded it as a sacred object and would hardly allow me to touch it. He cried over it, and after it was framed had it put up in his room as a kind of ikon. I told him that he must write to Her Royal Highness to thank her for her goodness. This he was pleased to do, as he was very fond of writing letters, never before in his life having had anyone to write to. I allowed the letter to be dispatched unedited. It began 'My dear Princess' and ended 'Yours very sincerely'. Unorthodox as it was it was expressed in terms any courtier would have envied.

Other ladies followed the Queen's gracious example and sent their photographs to this delighted creature who had been all his life despised and rejected of men. His mantelpiece and table became so covered with photographs of handsome ladies, with dainty knicknacks and pretty trifles that they may almost have befitted the apartment of an Adonislike actor or of a famous tenor.

Through all these bewildering incidents and through the glamour of this great change Merrick still remained in many ways a mere child. He had all the invention of an imaginative boy or girl, the same love of 'make-believe', the same instinct of 'dressing up' and of personating heroic and impressive characters. This attitude of mind was illustrated by the following incident. Benevolent visitors had given me, from time to time, sums of money to be expended for the comfort of the *ci-devant* Elephant Man. When one Christmas was approaching I asked Merrick what he would like me to purchase as a Christmas present. He rather startled me by saying shyly that he would like a dressing-bag with silver fittings. He had seen a picture of such an article in an advertisement which he had furtively preserved.

The association of a silver-fitted dressing-bag with the poor wretch wrapped up in a dirty blanket in an empty shop was hard to comprehend. I fathomed the mystery in time, for Merrick made little secret of the fancies that haunted his boyish brain. Just as a small girl with a tinsel coronet and a window curtain for a train will realize the conception of a countess on her way to court, so Merrick loved to imagine himself a dandy and a young man about town. Mentally, no doubt, he had frequently 'dressed up' for the part. He could 'make-believe' with great effect, but he wanted something to render his fancied character more realistic. Hence the jaunty bag which was to assume the function of the toy coronet and

21

the window curtain that could transform a mite with a pigtail into a countess.

As a theatrical 'property' the dressing-bag was ingenious, since there was little else to give substance to the transformation. Merrick could not wear the silk hat of the dandy nor, indeed, any kind of hat. He could not adapt his body to the trimly cut coat. His deformity was such that he could wear neither collar nor tie, while in association with his bulbous feet the young blood's patent leather shoe was unthinkable. What was there left to make up the character? A lady had given him a ring to wear on his undeformed hand, and a noble lord had presented him with a very stylish walking-stick. But these things, helpful as they were, were hardly sufficing.

The dressing-bag, however, was distinctive, was explanatory and entirely characteristic. So the bag was obtained and Merrick the Elephant Man became, in the seclusion of his chamber, the Piccadilly exquisite, the young spark, the gallant, the 'nut'. When I purchased the article I realized that as Merrick could never travel he could hardly want a dressing-bag. He could not use the silver-backed brushes and the comb because he had no hair to brush. The ivory-handled razors were useless because he could not shave. The deformity of his mouth rendered an ordinary toothbrush of no avail, and as his monstrous lips could not hold a cigarette the cigarette-case was a mockery. The silver shoe-horn would be of no service in the putting on of his ungainly slippers, while the hat-brush was quite unsuited to the peaked cap with its visor.

Still the bag was an emblem of the real swell and of the knockabout Don Juan of whom he had read. So every day Merrick laid out upon his table, with proud precision, the silver brushes, the razors, the show-horn and the silver cigarette-case which I had taken care to fill with cigarettes. The contemplation of these gave him great pleasure, and such is the power of self-deception that they convinced him he was the 'real thing'.

I think there was just one shadow in Merrick's life. As I have already said, he had a lively imagination; he was romantic; he cherished an emotional regard for women and his favourite pursuit was the reading of love stories. He fell in love – in a humble and devotional way – with, I think, every attractive lady he saw. He, no doubt, pictured himself the hero of many a passionate incident. His bodily deformity had left unmarred the instincts and feelings of his years. He was amorous. He would like to have been a lover, to have walked with the beloved object in the languorous shades of some beautiful garden and to have poured into her ear all the glowing utterances that he had rehearsed in his heart. And yet – the pity of it! – imagine the feelings of such a youth when he saw nothing but a look of horror creep over the face of every girl whose eyes met his. I fancy when he talked of life among the blind there was a half-formed idea in his mind that he might be able to win the affection of a woman if only she were without eyes to see.

As Merrick developed he began to display certain modest ambitions in the direction of improving his mind and enlarging his knowledge of the world. He was as curious as a child and as eager to learn. There were so many things he wanted to know and to see. In the first place he was anxious to view the interior of what he called 'a real house', such a house as figured in many of the tales he knew, a house with a hall, a drawing-room where guests were received and a dining-room with plate on the sideboard and with easy chairs into which the hero could 'fling himself'. The workhouse, the common lodging-house and a variety of mean garrets were all the residences he knew. To satisfy this wish I drove him up to my small house in Wimpole Street. He was absurdly interested, and examined everything in detail and with untiring curiosity. I could not show him the pampered menials and the powdered footmen of whom he had read, nor could I produce the white marble staircase of the mansion of romance nor the gilded mirrors and the brocaded divans which belong to that style of residence. I explained that the house was a modest dwelling of the Jane Austen type, and as he had read 'Emma' he was content.

A more burning ambition of his was to go to the theatre. It

was a project very difficult to satisfy. A popular pantomime was then in progress at Drury Lane Theatre, but the problem was how so conspicuous a being as the Elephant Man could be got there, and how he was to see the performance without attracting the notice of the audience and causing a panic or, at least, an unpleasant diversion. The whole matter was most ingeniously carried through by that kindest of women and most able of actresses – Mrs. Kendal. She made the necessary arrangements with the lessee of the theatre. A box was obtained. Merrick was brought up in a carriage with drawn blinds and was allowed to make use of the royal entrance so as to reach the box by a private stair. I had begged three of the hospital sisters to don evening dress and to sit in the front row in order to 'dress' the box, on the one hand, and to form a screen for Merrick on the other. Merrick and I occupied the back of the box which was kept in shadow. All went well, and no one saw a figure, more monstrous than any on the stage, mount the staircase or cross the corridor.

One has often witnessed the unconstrained delight of a child at its first pantomime, but Merrick's rapture was much more intense as well as much more solemn. Here was a being with the brain of a man, the fancies of a youth and the imagination of a child. His attitude was not so much that of delight as of wonder and amazement. He was awed. He was enthralled. The spectacle left him speechless, so that if he were spoken to he took no heed. He often seemed to be panting for breath. I could not help comparing him with a man of his own age in the stalls. This satiated individual was bored to distraction, would look wearily at the stage from time to time and then yawn as if he had not slept for nights; while at the same time Merrick was thrilled by a vision that was almost beyond his comprehension. Merrick talked of this pantomime for weeks and weeks. To him, as to a child with the faculty of make-believe, everything was real; the palace was the home of kings, the princess was of royal blood, the fairies were as undoubted as the children in the street, while the dishes at the banquet were of unquestionable gold. He did not like to discuss it as a play but rather as a vision of some actual world. When this mood possessed him he would say: 'I wonder what the prince did after we left,' or 'Do you think that poor man is still in the dungeon?' and so on and so on.

The splendour and display impressed him, but, I think, the ladies of the ballet took a still greater hold upon his fancy. He did not like the ogres and the giants, while the funny men impressed him as irreverent. Having no experience as a boy of romping and ragging, of practical jokes or of 'larks', he had little sympathy with the doings of the clown, but, I think (moved by some mischievous instinct in his subconscious mind), he was pleased when the policeman was smacked in the face, knocked down and generally rendered undignified.

Later on another longing stirred the depths of Merrick's mind. It was a desire to see the country, a desire to live in some green secluded spot and there learn something about flowers and the ways of animals and birds. The country as viewed from a wagon on a dusty high road was all the country he knew. He had never wandered among the fields nor followed the windings of a wood. He had never climbed to the brow of a breezy down. He had never gathered flowers in a meadow. Since so much of his reading dealt with country life he was possessed by the wish to see the wonders of that life himself.

This involved a difficulty greater than that presented by a visit to the theatre. The project was, however, made possible on this occasion also by the kindness and generosity of a lady – Lady Knightley – who offered Merrick a holiday home in a cottage on her estate. Merrick was conveyed to the railway station in the usual way, but as he could hardly venture to appear on the platform the railway authorities were good enough to run a second-class carriage into a distant siding. To this point Merrick was driven and was placed in the carriage unobserved. The carriage, with the curtains drawn, was then attached to the mainline train.

He duly arrived at the cottage, but the housewife (like the nurse at the hospital) had not been made clearly aware of the unfortunate man's appearance. Thus it happened that when

25

Merrick presented himself his hostess, throwing her apron over her head, fled, gasping, to the fields. She affirmed that such a guest was beyond her powers of endurance, for, when she saw him, she was 'that took' as to be in danger of being permanently 'all of a tremble'.

Merrick was then conveyed to a gamekeeper's cottage which was hidden from view and was close to the margin of a wood. The man and his wife were able to tolerate his presence. They treated him with the greatest kindness, and with them he spent the one supreme holiday of his life. He could roam where he pleased. He met no one on his wanderings, for the wood was preserved and denied to all but the gamekeeper and the forester.

There is no doubt that Merrick passed in this retreat the happiest time he had as yet experienced. He was alone in a land of wonders. The breath of the country passed over him like a healing wind. Into the silence of the wood the fearsome voice of the showman could never penetrate. No cruel eyes could peep at him through the friendly undergrowth. It seemed as if in this place of peace all stain had been wiped away from his sullied past. The Merrick who had once crouched terrified in the filthy shadows of a Mile End shop was now sitting in the sun, in a clearing among the trees, arranging a bunch of violets he had gathered.

His letters to me were the letters of a delighted and enthusiastic child. He gave an account of his trivial adventures, of the amazing things he had seen, and of the beautiful sounds he had heard. He had met with strange birds, had startled a hare from her form, had made friends with a fierce dog, and had watched the trout darting in a stream. He sent me some of the wild flowers he had picked. They were of the commonest and most familiar kind, but they were evidently regarded by him as rare and precious specimens.

He came back to London, to his quarters in Bedstead Square, much improved in health, pleased to be 'home' again and to be once more among his books, his treasures and his many friends.

Some six months after Merrick's return from the country

he was found dead in bed. This was in April, 1890. He was lying on his back as if asleep, and had evidently died suddenly and without a struggle, since not even the coverlet of the bed was disturbed. The method of his death was peculiar. So large and so heavy was his head that he could not sleep lying down. When he assumed the recumbent position the massive skull was inclined to drop backwards, with the result that he experienced no little distress. The attitude he was compelled to assume when he slept was very strange. He sat up in bed with his back supported by pillows, his knees were drawn up, and his arms clasped round his legs, while his head rested on the points of his bent knees.

He often said to me that he wished he could lie down to sleep 'like other people'. I think on this last night he must, with some determination, have made the experiment. The pillow was soft, and the head, when placed on it, must have fallen backwards and caused a dislocation of the neck. Thus it came about that his death was due to the desire that had dominated his life – the pathetic but hopeless desire to be 'like other people'.

As a specimen of humanity, Merrick was ignoble and repulsive; but the spirit of Merrick, if it could be seen in the form of the living, would assume the figure of an upstanding and heroic man, smooth browed and clean of limb, and with eyes that flashed undaunted courage.

His tortured journey had come to an end. All the way he, like another, had borne on his back a burden almost too grievous to bear. He had been plunged into the Slough of Despond, but with manly steps had gained the farther shore. He had been made 'a spectacle to all men' in the heartless streets of Vanity Fair. He had been ill-treated and reviled and bespattered with the mud of Disdain. He had escaped the clutches of the Giant Despair, and at last had reached the 'Place of Deliverance', where 'his burden loosed from off his shoulders and fell from off his back, so that he saw it no more'.

*　　*　　*

From *The Times*, December 4, 1886

To the Editor of the Times

Sir, – I am authorized to ask your powerful assistance in bringing to the notice of the public the following most exceptional case. There is now in a little room off one of our attic wards a man named Joseph Merrick, aged about 27, a native of Leicester, so dreadful a sight that he is unable even to come out by daylight to the garden. He has been called 'the elephant man' on account of his terrible deformity. I will not shock your readers with any detailed description of his infirmities, but only one arm is available for work.

Some 18 months ago, Mr. Treves, one of the surgeons of the London Hospital, saw him as he was exhibited in a room off the Whitechapel-road. The poor fellow was then covered by an old curtain, endeavouring to warm himself over a brick which was heated by a lamp. As soon as a sufficient number of pennies had been collected by the manager at the door, poor Merrick threw off his curtain and exhibited himself in all his deformity. He and the manager went halves in the net proceeds of his exhibition, until at last the police stopped the exhibition of his deformities as against public decency. Unable to earn his livelihood by exhibiting himself any longer in England, he was persuaded to go over to Belgium, where he was taken in hand by an Austrian, who acted as his manager. Merrick managed in this way to save a sum of nearly £50, but the police there too kept him moving on, so that his life was a miserable and hunted one. One day, however, when the Austrian saw that the exhibition was pretty well played out, he decamped with poor Merrick's hardly-saved capital of £50, and left him alone and absolutely destitute in a foreign country. Fortunately, however, he had

28

something to pawn, by which he raised sufficient money to pay his passage back to England, for he felt that the only friend he had in the world was Mr. Treves, of the London Hospital. He therefore, though with much difficulty, made his way there, for at every station and landing-place the curious crowd so thronged and dogged his steps that it was not an easy matter for him to get about. When he reached the London Hospital he had only the clothes in which he stood. He has been taken in by our hospital, though there is, unfortunately, no hope of his cure, and the question now arises what is to be done with him in the future.

He has the greatest horror of the workhouse, nor is it possible, indeed, to send him into any place where he could not insure privacy, since his appearance is such that all shrink from him.

The Royal Hospital for Incurables and the British Home for Incurables both decline to take him in, even if sufficient funds were forthcoming to pay for him.

The police rightly prevent his being personally exhibited again; he cannot go out into the streets, as he is everywhere so mobbed that existence is impossible; he cannot, in justice to others, be put in the general ward of a workhouse, and from such, even if possible, he shrinks with the greatest horror; he ought not to be detained in our hospital (where he is occupying a private ward, and being treated with the greatest kindness – he says he has never before known in his life what quiet and rest were), since his case is incurable, and not suited, therefore, to our overcrowded general hospital; the incurable hospitals refuse to take him in even if we paid for him in full, and the difficult question therefore remains what is to be done for him.

Terrible though his appearance is, so terrible indeed that women and nervous persons fly in terror from the sight of him, and that he is debarred from seeking to earn his livelihood in any ordinary way, yet he is superior in intelligence, can read and write, is quiet, gentle, not to say even refined in his mind. He occupies his time in the hospital by making with his one available hand little cardboard models, which he sends to the matron, doctor, and those who have been kind to him. Through all the miserable vicissitudes of his life he has carried about a painting of his mother to show that she was a decent and presentable person, and as a memorial of the only one who was kind to him in life until he came under the kind care of the nursing staff of the London Hospital and the surgeon who has befriended him.

It is a case of singular affliction brought about through no fault of himself; he can but hope for quiet and privacy during a life which Mr. Treves assures me is not likely to be long.

Can any of your readers suggest to me some fitting place where he can be received? And then I feel sure that, when that is found, charitable people will come forward and enable me to provide him with such accommodation. In the meantime, though it is not the proper place for such an incurable case, the little room under the roof of our hospital and out of Cotton Ward supplies him with all he wants. The Master of the Temple on Advent Sunday preached an eloquent sermon on the subject of our Master's answer to the question, 'Who did sin, this man or his parents, that he was born blind?' showing how one of the Creator's objects in permitting men to be born to a life of hopeless and miserable disability was that the works of God should be manifested in evoking the sympathy and kindly aid of those on whom such a heavy cross is not laid.

Some 76,000 patients a year pass through the doors of our hospital, but I have never before been authorized to invite public attention to any particular case, so it may well be believed that this case is exceptional.

Any communication about this should be addressed either to myself or to the secretary at the London Hospital.

I have the honour to be, Sir, yours obediently,

    F.C. CARR GOMM, Chairman London Hospital.
November 30.

*   *   *

From *The Times*, April 16, 1890

To the Editor of the Times

Sir, – In November, 1886, you were kind enough to insert in
The Times a letter from me drawing attention to the case of
Joseph Merrick, known as 'the elephant man.' It was one of
singular and exceptional misfortune; his physical deformities
were of so appalling a character that he was debarred from
earning his livelihood in any other way than by being exhibited to the gaze of the curious. This having been rightly
interfered with by the police of this country, he was taken
abroad by an Austrian adventurer, and exhibited at different
places on the Continent; but one day his exhibitor, after
stealing all the savings poor Merrick had carefully hoarded,
decamped, leaving him destitute, friendless, and powerless
in a foreign country.

With great difficulty he succeeded somehow or other in
getting to the door of the London Hospital, where, through
the kindness of one of our surgeons, he was sheltered for a
time. The difficulty then arose as to his future; no incurable
hospital would take him in, he had a horror of the workhouse, and no place where privacy was unattainable was to be
thought of, while the rules and necessities of our general
hospital forbade the fund and space, which are set apart
solely for cure and healing, being utilized for the mainte-
nance of a chronic case like this, however abnormal. In this
dilemma, while deterred by common humanity from evicting
him again into the open street, I wrote to you, and from that
moment all difficulty vanished; the sympathy of many was
aroused, and, although no other fitting refuge offered, a
sufficient sum was placed at my disposal, apart from the
funds of the hospital, to maintain him for what did not
promise to be a prolonged life. As an exceptional case the
committee agreed to allow him to remain in the hospital upon

the annual payment of a sum equivalent to the average cost of an occupied bed.

Here, therefore, poor Merrick was enabled to pass the three and a half remaining years of his life in privacy and comfort. The authorities of the hospital, the medical staff, the chaplain, the sisters, and nurses united to alleviate as far as possible the misery of his existence, and he learnt to speak of his rooms at the hospital as his home. There he received kindly visits from many, among them the highest in the land, and his life was not without various interests and diversions: he was a great reader and was well supplied with books; through the kindness of a lady, one of the brightest ornaments of the theatrical profession, he was taught basket making, and on more than one occasion he was taken to the play, which he witnessed from the seclusion of a private box.

He benefited much from the religious instruction of our chaplain, and Dr. Walsham How, then Bishop of Bedford, privately confirmed him, and he was able by waiting in the vestry to hear and take part in the chapel services. The present chaplain tells me that on this Easter day, only five days before his death, Merrick was twice thus attending the chapel services, and in the morning partook of the Holy Communion; and in the last conversation he had with him Merrick had expressed his feeling of deep gratitude for all that had been done for him here, and his acknowledgment of the mercy of God to him in bringing him to this place. Each year he much enjoyed a six weeks' outing in a quiet country cottage, but was always glad on his return to find himself once more 'at home.' In spite of all this indulgence he was quiet and unassuming, very grateful for all that was done for him, and conformed himself readily to the restrictions which were necessary.

I have given these details, thinking that those who sent money to use for his support would like to know how their charity was applied. Last Friday afternoon, though apparently in his usual health, he quietly passed away in sleep.

I have left in my hands a small balance of the money which has been sent to me from time to time for his support, and this I now propose, after paying certain gratuities, to hand over to the general funds of the hospital. This course, I believe, will be consonant with the wishes of the contributors.

It was the courtesy of *The Times* in inserting my letter in 1886 that procured for this afflicted man a comfortable protection during the last years of a previously wretched existence, and I desire to take this opportunity of thankfully acknowledging it.

I am, Sir, your obedient servant,

F. C. CARR GOMM.

House Committee Room, London Hospital, April 15.

THE OLD RECEIVING ROOM

A house surgeon at a great accident hospital in the east of London happens upon strange scenes, some pathetic, some merely sordid, together with fragments of tragedy in which the most elemental passions and emotions of humanity are displayed. The chief place in which this experience is gained is the Receiving Room. I speak of a hospital not as it is now, but as it was some fifty years ago. The Receiving Room is a bare hall, painted stone colour. It contains as furniture rows of deal benches and as wall decoration a printed notice, framed and glazed, detailing vivid measures for restoring the apparently drowned. Below this helpful document is fixed an iron-bound money-box. There is, moreover, a long desk in the hall where entries are made and certificates and other papers issued. As a room for the reception of the sick and suffering it is a cold, harsh place, with about it an air of cynical indifference.

This hall serves as a waiting-room, and there are nearly always some people waiting in it. It may be a sniffing woman who has called for her dead husband's clothes. It may be a still breathless messenger with a 'midwifery card' in her hand, or a girl waiting for a dose of emergency medicine. There may be some minor accident cases also, such as a torn finger, a black eye like a bursting plum, a child who has swallowed a halfpenny, and a woman who has been 'knocked about cruel,' but has little to show for it except a noisy desire to have her husband 'locked up.' In certain days of stress, as on Saturday nights, when the air is heavy with alcohol, or on the occasion of a 'big' dock accident, the waiting-room is crowded with excited folk, with patients waiting their turn to be dressed, with policemen, busybodies, reporters and friends of the injured.

On each side of the waiting-hall is a dressing-room – one

for women, one for men. Into these rooms the accident cases are taken one after the other. Here the house surgeon and his dressers are engaged, and here the many-sided drama of the Receiving Room reaches its culminating point. It is an uninviting room, very plain, and, like the outer hall, bears an aspect of callous unconcern. By the window is a suspiciously large sink, and on the ledge above it a number of pewter porringers. One side of the room is occupied by a mysterious cupboard containing dressings, gags, manacles, emetics and other unattractive things. In the centre are a common table and two hard chairs.

The most repellent thing in the room is a low sofa. It is wide and is covered with very thick leather which is suspiciously shiny and black. It suggests no more comfort than a rack. Its associations are unpleasant. It has been smothered with blood and with every kind of imaginable filth, and has been cleaned up so often that it is no wonder that the deeply stained leather is shiny. It is on this grim black couch that 'the case' just carried into the hospital is placed. It may be a man ridden over in the street, with the red bone-ends of his broken legs sticking through his trousers. It may be a machine accident, where strips of cotton shirt have become tangled up with torn flesh and a trail of black grease. It may be a man picked up in a lane with his throat cut, or a woman, dripping foul mud, who has been dragged out of a river. Sometimes the occupant of the sofa is a snoring lump of humanity so drunk as to be nearly dead, or it may be a panting woman who has taken poison and regretted it. In both cases the stomach pump is used with nauseating incidents. Now and then the sofa is occupied by a purple-faced maniac, who is pinned down by sturdy dressers while a straitjacket is being applied to him. This is not the whole of its history nor of its services, for the Receiving Room nurse, who is rather proud of it, likes to record that many a man and many a woman have breathed their last on this horrible divan.

The so-called dressing room is at its best a 'messy' place, as two mops kept in the corner seem to suggest. It is also at times a noisy place, since the yells and screams that escape from it may be heard in the street and may cause passers-by to stop and look up at the window.

Among the sick and the maimed who are 'received' in this unsympathetic hall, the most pathetic are the wondering babies and the children. Many are brought in burnt and wrapped up in blankets, with only their singed hair showing out of the bundle. Others have been scalded, so that tissue-paper-like sheets of skin come off when their dressings are applied. Not a few, in old days, were scalded in the throat from drinking out of kettles. Then there are the children who have swallowed things, and who have added to the astounding collection of articles – from buttons to prayer-book clasps – which have found their way, at one time or another, into the infant interior, as well as children who have needles embedded in parts of their bodies or have been bitten by dogs or cats or even by rats.

I remember one bloated, half-dressed woman who ran screaming into the Receiving Room with a dead baby in her arms. She had gone to bed drunk, and had awakened in the morning in a tremulous state to find a dead infant by her side. This particular experience was not unusual in Whitechapel. Then there was another woman who rushed in drawing attention to a thing like a tiny bead of glass sticking to her baby's cheek. The child had acute inflammation of the eyeball, which the mother had treated with cold tea. The eye had long been closed, but when the mother made a clumsy attempt to open the swollen lids something had popped out, some fluid and this thing like glass. She was afraid to touch it. She viewed it with horror as a strange thing that had come out of the eye. Hugging the child, she had run a mile or so with the dread object still adhering to the skin of the cheek. This glistening thing was the crystalline lens. The globe had been burst, and the child was, of course, blind. Happily, such a case could hardly be met with at the present day.

On the subject of children and domestic surgery as revealed in the Receiving Room, I recall the case of a boy aged about four who had pushed a dry pea into his ear. The mother attempted to remove it with that common surgical implement of the home, a hairpin. She not only failed, but succeeded in pushing the pea farther down into the bony part of the canal. Being a determined woman, she borrowed a squirt, and proceeded to syringe out the foreign body with hot water. The result was that the pea swelled, and, being encased in bone, caused so intense and terrible a pain that the boy became unconscious from shock.

Possibly the most dramatic spectacle in connexion with Receiving Room life in pre-ambulance days was the approach to the hospital gate of a party carrying a wounded woman or man. Looking out of the Receiving Room window on such occasion a silent crowd would be seen coming down the street. It is a closely packed crowd which moves like a clot, which occupies the whole pavement and oozes over into the road. In the centre of the mass is an obscure object towards which all eyes are directed. In the procession are many women, mostly with tousled heads, men, mostly without caps, a butcher, a barber's assistant, a trim postman, a whitewasher, a man in a tall hat, and a pattering fringe of ragged boys. The boys, being small, cannot see much, so they race ahead in relays to glimpse the fascinating object from the front or climb up railings or mount upon steps to get a view of it as it passes by. Possibly towering above the throng would be two policemen, presenting an air of assumed calm; but policemen were not so common in those days as they are now.

The object carried would be indistinct, being hidden from view as is the queen bee by a clump of fussing bees. Very often the injured person is merely carried along by hand, like a parcel that is coming to pieces. There would be a man to each leg and to each arm, while men on either side would hang on to the coat. Possibly some Samaritan, walking backwards, would hold up the dangling head. It was a much prized distinction to clutch even a fragment of the sufferer or to carry his hat or the tools he had dropped.

At this period the present-day stretcher was unknown in civil life. A stretcher provided by the docks was a huge structure with high sides. It was painted green, and was solid enough to carry a horse. A common means of conveyance for the helpless was a shutter, but with the appearance of the modern ambulance the shutter has become as out of date as the sedan chair. Still, at this time, when anyone was knocked down in the street some bright, resourceful bystander would be sure to call out 'Send for a shutter!'

The conveying of a drunken man with a cut head to the hospital by the police (in the ancient fashion) was a more hilarious ceremonial. The 'patient' would be hooked up on either side by an official arm. His body would sag between these two supports so that his shoulders would be above his ears. His clothes would be worked up in folds about his neck, and he would appear to be in danger of slipping earthwards out of them. As it was, there would be a display of shirt and braces very evident below his coat. His legs would dangle below him like roots, while his feet, as they dragged along the pavement, would be twisted now in one direction and now in another like the feet of a badly stuffed lay figure. He would probably be singing as he passed along, to the delight of the people.

Of the many Receiving Room processions that I have witnessed the most moving, the most savage and the most rich in colour, noise and language was on an occasion when two 'ladies' who had been badly lacerated in a fight were being dragged, carried or pushed towards the hospital for treatment. They were large, copious women who were both in an advanced stage of intoxication. They had been fighting with gin bottles in some stagnent court which had become, for the moment, an uproarious cockpit. The technique of such a duel is punctilious. The round, smooth bottoms of the bottles are knocked off, and the combatants, grasping the weapons by the neck, proceed to jab one another in the face with the jagged circles of broken glass.

The wounds in this instance were terrific. The faces of the two, hideously distorted, were streaming with blood, while their ample bodies seemed to have been drenched with the same. Their hair, soaked in blood, was plastered to their heads like claret-coloured seaweed on a rock. The two heroines were borne along by their women friends. The police kept wisely in the background, for their time was not yet. The crowd around the two bleeding figures was so compressed that the whole mass moved as one. It was a wild crowd, a writhing knot of viragoes who roared and screamed and rent the air with curses and yells of vengeance, for they were partisans in the fight, the Montagues and Capulets of a ferocious feud.

The crowd as it came along rocked to and fro, heaved and lurched as if propelled by some uneasy sea. The very pavement seemed unsteady. Borne on the crest of this ill-smelling wave were the two horrible women. One still shrieked threats and defiance in a voice as husky as that of a beast, while now and then she lifted aloft a blood-streaked arm in the hand of which was clutched a tuft of hair torn from her opponent's head. Every display of this trophy called forth a shout of pride from her admirers.

The other woman was in a state of drunken hysteria. Throwing back her head until the sun illumined her awful features, she gave vent to bursts of maniacal laughter which were made peculiarly hideous by the fact that her nose was nearly severed from her face, while her grinning lips were hacked in two. At another moment, burying her head against the back of the woman in front of her, she would break out into sobs and groans which were even more unearthly than her laughter.

The whole affair suggested some fearful Bacchanalian orgy, associated with bloodshed, in which all concerned were the subjects of demoniacal possession. There is happily, much less drunkenness nowadays and less savagery, while the police control of these 'street scenes' is so efficient and the public ambulance so secretive that such a spectacle as I now recall belongs for ever to the past.

When a crowd, bearing a 'casualty,' reaches the hospital gates its progress is stayed. It rolls up against the iron barrier. It stops and recoils like a muddy wave against a bank. The porter is strict. Only the principals, their supporters and the police are allowed to filter through. The members of the crowd remain in the street, where they look through the railings, to which they cling, and indulge in fragments of narrative, in comments on the affair, and on the prospects of the parties injured. If a scream should escape from the Receiving Room the watchers feel that they are well rewarded for long waiting, while any member of the privileged party who may leave the building is subjected to very earnest questioning.

It is needless to say that the Receiving Room is not always tragical, not always the scene of alarms and disorders, not always filled with wild-eyed folk nor echoing the scuffle of heavy feet and the moans of the suffering. It may be as quiet as a room in a convent. I have seen it so many a time, and particularly on a Sunday morning in the heyday of summer. Then the sun, streaming through the windows, may illumine the figure of the nurse as she sits on the awful sofa. She has her spectacles on, and is busy with some white needlework. Her attitude is so placid that she might be sitting at a cottage door listening to a blackbird in a wicker cage. Yet this quiet-looking woman, although she has not fought with wild beasts at Ephesus, has fought with raving drunkards and men delirious from their hurts, and has heard more foul language and more blasphemy in a week than would have enlivened a pirate ship in a year.

The Receiving Room nurse was, in old days, without exception the most remarkable woman in the hospital. She appeared as a short, fat, comfortable person of middle age, with a ruddy face and a decided look of assurance. She was without education, and yet her experience of casualties of all kinds – from a bee-sting to sudden death – was vast and indeed unique. She was entirely self-taught, for there were no trained nurses in those days. She was of the school of Mrs. Gamp, was a woman of courage and of infinite resource, an expert in the treatment of the violent and in the crushing of anyone who gave her what she called 'lip.' She was possessed of much humour, was coarse in her language, abrupt, yet not unkindly in her manner, very indulgent towards the drunk-

40

ard and very skilled in handling him. She was apt to boast that there was no man living she would not 'stand up to.' She called every male over fifty 'Daddy' and every one under that age 'My Son.' She would tackle a shrieking woman as a terrier tackles a rat, while the woman who 'sauced' her she soon reduced to a condition of palsy. She objected to the display of emotion or of feeling in any form, and was apt to speak of members of her sex as a 'watery-headed lot.'

She had, like most nurses of her time, a leaning towards gin, but was efficient even in her cups. She had wide powers, for she undertook – on her own responsibility – the treatment of petty casualties. The dressers regarded her with respect. Her knowledge and skill amazed them, while from her they acquired the elements of minor surgery and first aid. The house surgeons were a little frightened of her, yet they admired her ready craft and were duly grateful for her unswerving loyalty and her eagerness to save them trouble. Her diagnosis of an injury was probably correct, so sound was her observation and wide her experience. She was a brilliant bandager, and was accepted by the students as the standard of style and finish in the applying of a dressing. She was on duty from early in the morning until late at night, and knew little of 'hours off' and 'half-days.' In the personnel of the hospital of half a century ago she was an outstanding figure, yet now she is as extinct as the dodo.

The hospital in the days of which I speak was anathema. The poor people hated it. They dreaded it. They looked upon it primarily as a place where people died. It was a matter of difficulty to induce a patient to enter the wards. They feared an operation, and with good cause, for an operation then was a very dubious matter. There were stories afloat of things that happened in the hospital, and it could not be gainsaid that certain of those stories were true.

Treatment was very rough. The surgeon was rough. He had inherited that attitude from the days when operations were carried through without anæsthetics, and when he had need to be rough, strong and quick, as well as very indifferent to pain. Pain was with him a thing that had to be. It was a

41

regrettable feature of disease. It had to be submitted to. At the present day pain is a thing that has not to be. It has to be relieved and not to be merely endured.

Many common measures of treatment involved great suffering. Bleeding was still a frequent procedure, and to the timid the sight of the red stream trickling into the bowl was a spectacle of terror. There were two still more common measures in use – the seton and the issue. The modern student knows nothing of these ancient and uncleanly practices. He must inform himself by consulting a dictionary. Without touching upon details, I may say that in my early days, as a junior dresser, one special duty was to run round the ward before the surgeon arrived in order to draw a fresh strand of thread through each seton and to see that a fresh pea was forced into the slough of every issue.

Quite mediæval methods were still observed. The first time in my life that I saw the interior of an operating theatre I, in my ignorance, entered by the door which opened directly into the area where the operating table stood. (I should have entered by the students' gallery.) When I found myself in this amazing place there was a man on the table who was shrieking vehemently. The surgeon, taking me by the arm, said, 'You seem to have a strong back; lay hold of that rope and pull.' I laid hold of the rope. There were already two men in front of me and we all three pulled our best. I had no idea what we were pulling for. I was afterwards informed that the operation in progress was the reduction of a dislocated hip by compound pulleys. The hip, however, was not reduced and the man remained lame for life. At the present day a well-instructed schoolgirl could reduce a recent hip dislocation unaided.

In this theatre was a stove which was always kept alight, winter and summer, night and day. The object was to have a fire at all times ready whereat to heat the irons used for the arrest of bleeding as had been the practice since the days of Elizabeth. Antiseptics were not yet in use. Sepsis was the prevailing condition in the wards. Practically all major wounds suppurated. Pus was the most common subject of converse, because it was the most prominent feature in the surgeon's work. It was classified according to degrees of vileness. 'Laudable' pus was considered rather a fine thing, something to be proud of. 'Sanious' pus was not only nasty in appearance but regrettable, while 'ichorous' pus represented the most malignant depths to which matter could attain.

There was no object in being clean. Indeed, cleanliness was out of place. It was considered to be finicking and affected. An executioner might as well manicure his nails before chopping off a head. The surgeon operated in a slaughter-house-suggesting frock coat of black cloth. It was stiff with the blood and the filth of years. The more sodden it was the more forcibly did it bear evidence to the surgeon's prowess. I, of course, commenced my surgical career in such a coat, of which I was quite proud. Wounds were dressed with 'charpie' soaked in oil. Both oil and dressing were frankly and exultingly septic. Charpie was a species of cotton waste obtained from cast linen. It would probably now be discarded by a motor mechanic as being too dirty for use on a car.

Owing to the suppurating wounds the stench in the wards was of a kind not easily forgotten. I can recall it to this day with unappreciated ease. There was one sponge to a ward. With this putrid article and a basin of once-clear water all the wounds in the ward were washed in turn twice a day. By this ritual any chance that a patient had of recovery was eliminated. I remember a whole ward being decimated by hospital gangrene. The modern student has no knowledge of this disease. He has never seen it and, thank heaven, he never will. People often say how wonderful it was that surgical patients lived in these days. As a matter of fact they did not live, or at least only a few of them. Lord Roberts assured me that on the Ridge at Delhi during the Indian Mutiny no case of amputation recovered. This is an extreme instance, for the conditions under which the surgeons on the Ridge operated were exceptional and hopelessly unfavourable.

The attitude that the public assumed towards hospitals and their works at the time of which I write may be illustrated by the following incident. I was instructed by my surgeon to obtain a woman's permission for an operation on her daughter. The operation was one of no great magnitude. I interviewed the mother in the Receiving Room. I discussed the procedure with her in great detail and, I trust, in a sympathetic and hopeful manner. After I had finished my discourse I asked her if she would consent to the performance of the operation. She replied: 'Oh! it is all very well to talk about consenting, but who is to pay for the funeral?'

THE TWENTY-KRONE PIECE

More than once in speaking at public meetings on behalf of hospitals I have alluded to my much valued possession – a twenty-krone piece – and have employed it as an illustration of the gratitude of the hospital patient.

The subject of this incident was a Norwegian sailor about fifty years of age, a tall, good-featured man with the blue eyes of his country and a face tanned by sun and by salt winds to the colour of weathered oak. His hair and his beard were grey, which made him look older than he was. He had been serving for three years as an ordinary seaman on an English sailing ship and spoke English perfectly. During his last voyage he had developed a trouble which prevented him from following his employment. Accordingly he had left his ship and made his way to London in the hope of being cured. Inquiring for the hospital of London he was directed to the London Hospital and, by chance, came into my wards. He had an idea – as I was told later – that the operation he must needs undergo might be fatal, and so had transferred his savings to his wife in Norway.

He was a quiet and reserved man, but so pleasant in his manner that he became a favourite with the nurses. He told them quaintly-worded tales of his adventures and showed them how to make strange knots with bandages. The operation – which was a very ordinary one – was successful, and in four or five weeks he was discharged as capable of resuming his work as a seaman. His ship had, however, long since started on another voyage.

One morning, three weeks after he had left the hospital, he appeared at my house in Wimpole Street. My name he would have acquired from the board above his bed, but I wondered how he had obtained my address. I assumed that he had called to ask for money or for help of some kind. As he came into my room I was sorry to see how thin and ill he looked, for when he left the wards he was well and hearty.

He proceeded to thank me for what I had done, little as it was. He had an exaggerated idea of the magnitude of the operation, which idea he would not allow me to correct. I have listened to many votes of thanks, to the effulgent language, the gush and the pompous flattery which have marked them; but the little speech of this sailor man was not of that kind. It was eloquent by reason of its boyish simplicity, its warmth and its rugged earnestness.

As he was speaking he drew from his pocket a gold coin, a twenty-krone piece, and placed it on the table at which I sat. 'I beg you, sir,' he said, 'to accept this coin. I know it is of no value to you. It is only worth, I think, fifteen shillings. It would be an insult to offer it as a return for what you have done for me. That service can never be repaid. But I hope you will accept it as a token of what I feel, of something that I cannot say in words but that this coin can tell of. When I left my home in Norway three years ago my wife sewed this twenty-krone piece in the band of my trousers and made me promise never to touch it until I was starving. A seaman's life is uncertain; he may be ill, he may be long out of a job; and so for three years this coin has been between me and the risk of starvation. When I was in the hospital I had a wish to give it to you if it so happened that I got well. Here I am, and I do hope, sir, you will accept it.'

I thanked him as warmly as I could for his kindness, for his thought in coming to see me and for his touching offer, but added that I could not possibly take the gold piece and begged him to put it back into his pocket again and present it to his wife when he reached home. At this he was very much upset. Pushing the coin along the table towards me with his forefinger, he said: 'Please, sir, do take the money, not for what it is worth but for what it has been to me. I am proud to say that since I left the hospital I *have* been starving. I have been looking for a ship. I have not slept in a bed since you saw me in the wards. Now, at last, I have got a ship and, thank

God, I have kept the coin unbroken so that you might have it. I implore you to accept it.'

I took it; but what could I say that would be adequate for such a gift as this? My attempt at thanks was as stumbling and as feeble as his had been outright; for I am not ashamed to confess that I was much upset.

I have received many presents from kindly patients – silver bowls, diamond scarf-pins, gold cigarette cases and the like, but how little is their value compared with this one small coin? As I picked it up from the table I thought of what it had cost. I thought of the tired man haunting the docks in search of a ship, often aching with hunger and at night sleeping in a shed, and yet all the time with a piece of gold in his pocket which he would not change in order that I might have it.

A coin is an emblem of wealth, but this gold piece is an emblem of a rarer currency, of that wealth which is – in a peculiar sense – 'beyond the dream of avarice,' a something that no money could buy, for what sum could express the bounty or the sentiment of this generous heart?

It would be described, by those ignorant of its history, as a gold coin from Norway; but I prefer to think that it belongs to that 'land of Havilah where there is gold' and of which it is truly said 'and the gold of that land is good.'

A CURE FOR NERVES

In the account of the case which follows it is better that I allow the patient to speak for herself.

I am a neurotic woman. In that capacity I have been the subject of much criticism and much counsel. I have been both talked to and talked at. On the other hand I have detailed my unhappy symptoms to many in the hope of securing consolation, but with indefinite success. I am afraid I have often been a bore; for a bore, I am told, is a person who will talk of herself when you want to talk of yourself.

My husband says that there is nothing the matter with me, that my ailments are all imaginary and unreasonable. He becomes very cross when I talk of my wretched state and considers my ill-health as a grievance personal to himself. He says – when he is very irritated – that he is sick of my moanings, that I look well, eat well, sleep well, and so must be as sound as a woman can be. If I have a headache and cannot go out he is more annoyed than if he had the headache himself, which seems to me irrational. He is often very sarcastic about my symptoms, and this makes me worse. Once or twice he has been sympathetic and I have felt better, but he says that sympathy will do me harm and cause me to give way more. I suppose he knows because he is always so certain. He says all I have to do is to cheer up, to rouse myself, to pull myself together. He slaps himself on the chest and, in a voice that makes my head crack, says, 'Look at me! I am not nervous, why should you be?' I don't know why I am nervous and so I never try to answer the question. From the way my husband talks I feel that he must regard me as an impostor. If we have a few friends to dinner he is sure to say something about 'the deplorable flabbiness of the minds of some women.' I know he is addressing himself to me and so do the others, but I can only smile and feel uncomfortable.

I have no wish to be nervous. It is miserable enough, heaven knows. I would give worlds to be free of all my miseries and be quite sound again. If I wished to adopt a complaint I should choose one less hideously distressing than 'nerves.' I have often thought I would sooner be blind than nervous, and that then my husband would be really sorry for me; but I should be terribly frightened to be always in the dark.

I get a good deal of comfort from many of my women friends. They at least are sympathetic; they believe in me, know that my complaints are real and that what I say is true. Unfortunately, when I have described certain of my symptoms – such as one of my gasping attacks – they say that they have just such attacks themselves, only worse. They are so sorry for me; but then they will go on and tell me the exact circumstances under which they have had their last bouts. I am anxious to tell them of my other curious symptoms, but they say that it does them so much good to pour out their hearts to someone, and I, being very meek, let them go on, only wishing that they would listen to me as I listen to them.

I notice that their husbands have for the most part just the same erroneous views about nerves that mine has. Some of them say that they would like to make their menfolk suffer as they do themselves. One lady I know always ends with the reflection: 'Ah, well! I shall not be long here, and when I am dead and under the daisies he will be sorry he was not more appreciative. He will then know, when it is too late, that my symptoms were genuine enough.' I must say that I have never gone to the extreme of wishing to die for the mere sake of convincing my husband of obstinate stupidity. I should like to go into a death-like trance and frighten him, for then I should be able to hear what he said when he thought I was gone and remind him of it afterwards whenever he became cynical.

It is in the morning that I feel so bad. I am really ghastly then. I wake up with the awful presentiment that something dreadful is going to happen. I don't know what it is, yet I feel I could sink through the bed. I imagine the waking moments

49

of the poor wretch who has been condemned to death and who is said to have 'slept well' on the night before his execution. He will probably awake slowly and will feel at first hazily happy and content, will yawn and smile, until there creeps up the horrible recollection of the judge and the sentence, of the gallows and the hanging by the neck. I know the cold sweat that breaks over the whole body and the sickly clutching about the heart that attend such an awakening, but doubt if any emerging from sleep can be really worse than many I have experienced.

I can do so little in the day-time. I soon get exhausted and so utterly done up that I can only lie still in a dark room. When I am like that the least noise worries me and even tortures me almost out of my mind. If someone starts strumming the piano, or if a servant persistently walks about with creaky boots, or if my husband bursts in and tries to be hearty, I feel compelled to scream, it is so unbearable.

It is on such an occasion as this that my husband is apt to beg me 'to pull myself together.' He quite maddens me when he says this. I feel as full of terror, awfulness and distress as a drowning man, and how silly it would be to lean over a harbour wall and tell a drowning man in comfortable tones that he should 'pull himself together.' Yet that is what my husband says to me, with the irritating conviction that he is being intelligent and practical.

I cannot walk out alone. If I attempt it I am soon panic-stricken. I become hot all over, very faint, and so giddy that I reel and have to keep to the railings of the houses. I am seized with the hideous feeling that I can neither get on nor get back. I am not disturbed by the mere possibility of falling down on the pavement, but by the paralysing nightmare that I cannot take another step.

If anyone were to put me down in the middle of a great square, like the Praço de Dom Pedro at Lisbon, and leave me there alone, I think I should die or lose my reason. I know I should be unable to get out. I should fall in a heap, shut my eyes and try to crawl to the edge on my hands and knees, filled all the time with a panting terror. A man who finds himself compelled to cross a glassy ice slope which, twenty feet below, drops over a precipice, could not feel worse than I do if left adrift, nor pray more fervently to be clear of the abhorred space and safe. My husband says that this is all nonsense. I suppose it is, but it is such nonsense as would be sense if the jester were Death.

The knowledge that I have to go to a dinner party fills me with unutterable alarm. By the time I am dressed and ready to start I am chilled, shaking all over and gasping for breath. The drive to the house is almost as full of horror as the drive of the tumbril to the guillotine. By the time I arrive I am so ill I can hardly speak and am convinced that I shall fall down, or be sick, or shall have to cry out. More than once I have insisted upon being driven home again, and my husband has gone to the dinner alone after much outpouring of language.

Possibly my most direful experiments have been at the theatre, to which I have been taken on the ground that my mind needed change and that a cheerful play would 'take me out of myself.' My worst terrors have come upon me when I have chanced to sit in the centre of the stalls with people packed in all around me. I have then felt as if I was imprisoned and have been filled by one intense overwhelming desire – the passion to get out. I have passed through all the horrors of suffocation, have felt that I must stand up, must lift up my arms and gasp. I have looked at the door only to feel that escape was as impossible as it would be to an entrapped miner about whom the walls of a shaft had fallen.

It is useless for my husband to nudge me and tell me not to make a fool of myself. If I did want to make a fool of myself I should select some more agreeable way of doing it. It is useless, moreover, to argue. No argument can dispel the ever-present sense of panic, of being buried alive, or relieve the hopeless feeling of inability to escape. I have sat out a play undergoing tortures beyond expression, until I have become collapsed and until my lip had been almost bitten through in the effort not to scream. No one would believe that I – a healthy-looking woman in a new Paris dress, sitting among a company of smiling folk – could be enduring as much agony

51

as if I were lodged in an iron cell the walls of which were gradually closing in around me.

I am very fond of my clothes when I am well, but there are certain frocks I have come to loathe because they recall times when I have nearly gasped out my life in them.

I have taken much medicine but with no apparent good. I envy the woman who believes in her nerve tonic, since such faith must be a great comfort to her. I knew a poor girl who became for a time a mental wreck, owing to her engagement having been broken off. She refused food and lived for a week – so she told me – on her mother's nerve tonic. She declared that it saved her reason. I tried it, but it only brought me out in spots. I have seen a good many doctors, but although they are all very kind, they seem to be dense and to have but the one idea of treating the neurotic woman as they would treat a frightened child or a lost dog.

I was taken to one doctor because he had the reputation of being very sensible and outspoken. My husband said there was no nonsense about him. He certainly made no effort to be entertaining. After he had examined me he said that all my organs were perfectly sound. He then began to address me as 'My dear lady,' and at once I knew what was coming. It was to tell me that I wanted rousing and that all I had to do was to get out of myself. He said I was not to think about myself at all, which is very good advice to a person who feels on the point of dissolution. He told my husband afterwards, in strict confidence, that if I was a poor woman and had to work for my living I should be well directly. He went farther and said that what would cure me would be a week at the washing tub – at a laundry, I suppose. My husband imparted these confidences to me as we drove home from the doctor's and said what a shrewd, common-sense man he was. My husband quite liked him.

Another doctor I went to was very sympathetic. He patted my hand and was so kind that he almost made me cry. He said he understood how real and intense my sufferings were. He knew I must have gone through tortures. He gave me a great many particulars as to how I was to live and said I was never to do anything I did not like. I wanted to come and see him again, but he insisted that I must go abroad at once to break with my sad associations and afford my shattered nerves a complete rest. He gave me a letter to a doctor abroad which he said contained a very full and particular account of my case.

Something happened to prevent me from leaving England, but six months later I came across the letter and, feeling it was no longer of use, opened it. It began, 'My dear Harry,' and contained a great deal about their respective handicaps at golf and their plans for the summer. The kind doctor ended in this wise in a postscript: 'The lady who brings this is Mrs.—. She is a terrible woman, a deplorable neurotic. I need say no more about her, but I hope you won't mind my burdening you with her, for she is the kind of tedious person who bores me to death. However she pays her fees.' My husband sent the letter back to the doctor who wrote it, because he thought the memoranda about the golf handicaps would be interesting for him to keep.

As I made no progress and as my friends were getting as tired of me as I was of myself, it was resolved that I should be taken 'seriously in hand.' I was therefore sent to a nursing home to undergo the rest cure. I had to lie in bed, be stuffed with food and be massaged daily. I was cut off from all communion with the familiar world and was allowed to receive neither letters nor newspapers.

The idea underlying this measure is, I think, a little silly. It is in the main an attempt to cure a patient by enforced boredom. The inducement offered is crudely this: 'You can go home as soon as you think fit to be well.' I did not mind the quiet nor the lying in bed. The excessive feeding merely made me uncomfortable. The massage was a form of torture that I viewed with great loathing. The absence of news from home kept me in a state of unrest and apprehension. It was the continued speculation as to what was going on in my household which prevented me from sleeping at night.

The withdrawal of all newspapers was evidently a punishment devised by a man. It was no punishment to me nor would it be to the average woman. The nurse, of course, kept me informed of current events as she was extremely fond of talking and thereby rendered a newspaper unnecessary. She told me of the occasions when my husband called to inquire and always said that he looked very well and remarkably cheerful. She walked past my house once and came back with the information that the drawing-room blinds were up and that the sun was streaming into the room. This worried me a great deal as I don't like faded carpets and silks and am very fond of my furniture.

After I had been in the home a few days I discovered that the institution was not wholly devoted to rest-cure cases, but that it was also a surgical home where many operations were performed. This frightened me terribly because I began to wonder whether an operation had been an item of the programme when I was taken seriously in hand. I arrived at the conclusion that I was being 'prepared for operation,' that I was being 'built up,' with the result that I was prostrated by alarm. I felt that at any moment a man with a black bag might enter the room and proceed to chloroform me. There came upon me a conviction that I was being imprisoned, that I had been duped and trapped. Above all was the awful feeling, which nearly suffocated me, that I was powerless to escape. I thought my husband had been most base to desert me like this and hand me over, as it were, to unknown executioners.

I have a dread of operations which is beyond expression. The mere thinking of the process of being chloroformed makes me sick and faint. You are held down on a table, I believe, and then deliberately suffocated. It must be as if a man knelt upon your chest and strangled you by gripping your throat with his hands. When I was a small girl I saw a cook dispose of a live mouse by sinking the mouse-trap in which it was imprisoned in a bucket of water. I remember that the struggles of the mouse, as seen under water, were horrible to witness. When I grew up and was told about people being chloroformed for operation I always imagined that their feelings would be as hideous as those of the drowning mouse in a trap.

I told all my suspicions and alarms to the nurse, who laughed at me contemptuously. She said: 'You are merely a nerve case.' ('Merely,' thought I.) 'No surgeon ever thinks of operating on a nerve case. The greater number of the patients here come for very serious operations. They are real patients.' As she conversed further I must confess that my pride began to be touched. I had supposed that my case was the most important and most interesting in the establishment. I had the largest room in the house while the fussing over me had been considerable. I now began to learn that there were others who were in worse plight than myself. I, on the one hand, had merely to lie in bed and sleep. They, on the other, came to the home with their lives in their hands to confront an appalling ordeal. I was haunted by indefinite alarms; they had to submit to the tangible steel of the surgeon's knife. I began to be a little ashamed of myself and of the trouble I had occasioned. Compared with me these women were heroines. They had something to fuss about, for they had to walk alone into the Valley of the Shadow of Death. I had many times said that I wished I was dead, but a little reflection on the modes of dying made me keep that wish ever after unexpressed.

My nurse deplored that she was not a surgical nurse. 'To nurse an operation case is real nursing,' she said. 'There is something satisfactory in work like that. I am only a mental nurse, you see' – a confession which humbled me still further.

It was in September that I entered the home, and as the leading surgeons were still out of London there were no operations. When October came the gruesome work was resumed. The house was set vibrating with excitement. In this I shared as soon as I discovered that the operating theatre was immediately over my bedroom. Almost the first operation happened to be a particularly momentous one, concerned with which was none other than the great surgeon of the day. His coming was anticipated with a buzz of interest by the nurses, an interest which was even shared by the mental nurse in whose charge I was.

I could learn very little about this great case save that it was desperate and the victim a woman. I know that she entered the home the night before, for my nurse planned to meet her on her way to her room. I know also that just before the hour of closing the house I heard sobbing on the staircase as two people slowly made their way down. I came to know afterwards that one was the husband, the other the daughter.

The operation was to be at nine in the morning. By 6 A.M. the whole house was astir. There was much running up and down stairs. Everybody was occupied. My morning toilet and breakfast were hurried through with little ceremony. The nurse was excited, absent-minded and disinclined to answer questions. After my breakfast was cleared away she vanished – it was supposed that I was never to be left alone – and did not appear again until noon. When she did come back she found me an altered woman.

I lay in bed in the solitary room with my eyes fixed upon the white ceiling over my head. I was terrified beyond all reason. There was everywhere the sense of an overstrung activity, hushed and ominous, which was leading on to tragedy. I knew that in the room above me was about to be enacted a drama in which one of the actors was Death.

There was considerable bustle in the room in question. They were moving something very heavy into the middle of the floor. It was, I am sure, the operation table. Other tables were dragged about and adjusted with precision. Above the ceaseless patter of feet I could hear the pouring of water into basins.

I knew when the surgeon and his assistants arrived, for I heard his voice on the stair. It was clear and unconcerned, the one strong and confident thing among all these portentous preparations. Heavy bags were carried up from the hall to be deposited on the floor above. I could hear the surgeon's firm foot overhead and noticed a further moving of tables. There came now a clatter of steel in metal dishes which made me shiver.

I looked at the clock on my table. It was three minutes to nine.

What of the poor soul who was waiting? She also would be looking at the clock. Three minutes more and she would be led in her nightdress into this chamber of horrors. The very idea paralysed me. If I were in her place I should scream until I roused the street. I should struggle with every fibre of my body. I should cling to the door until my arms were pulled out of their sockets. A barrel-organ in the road was playing a trivial waltz, a boy was going by whistling, the world was cheerfully indifferent, while the loneliness of the stricken woman was horrible beyond words.

As the church clock struck nine I knew that the patient was entering the room. I fancied I could hear the shuffle of her slippers and the closing of the door – the last hope of escape – behind her. A chair was moved into position. She was stepping on to the table.

Then came an absolute silence. I knew they were chloroforming her. I fancied that the vapour of that sickly drug was oozing through the ceiling into my room. into my room. I was suffocated. I gasped until I thought my chest would burst. The silence was awful. I dared not scream. I would have rung my bell but the thought of the noise it would make held me back.

I lay glaring at the ceiling, my forehead covered with drops of cold sweat. I wrung my fingers together lest all sensation should go out of them.

In a while there came three awful moans from the room above and then once more the moving of feet was to be heard, whereby I felt that the operation had begun. I could picture the knife, the great cut, the cold callousness of it all. For what seemed to me to be interminable hours I gazed at the ceiling. How long was this murdering to go on! How could the poor moaning soul be tortured all this while and endure another minute!

Suddenly there was a great commotion in the room above. The table was dragged round rapidly. There were footsteps everywhere. Was the operation over? No. Something had gone wrong. A man dashed downstairs calling for a cab. In a moment I could hear the wheels tear along the street and then return. He had gone to fetch something and rushed upstairs with it.

This made me wonder for a moment what had happened to the husband and daughter who were waiting in a room off the hall. Had they died of the suspense? Why did they not burst into the room and drag her away while there was yet time? The lower part of the house was practically empty and I was conscious that two or three times the trembling couple had crept up the stairs to the level of my room to listen. I could hear the daughter say, 'What shall we do! What shall we do!' And then the two would stumble down the stairs again to the empty room.

I still glared at the ceiling like one in a trance. I had forgotten about myself, although there was such a sinking at my heart that I could only breathe in gasps. The loathsome bustle in the room above continued.

Now, as I gazed upwards, I noticed to my expressionless horror a small round patch of red appear on the white ceiling. I knew it was blood. The spot was as large as a five-shilling piece. It grew until it had become the size of a plate.

It burnt into my vision as if it had been a red-hot disk. It became a deeper crimson until at last one awful drop fell upon the white coverlet of my bed. It came down with the weight of lead. The impact went through me like an electric shock. I could hardly breathe. I was bathed with perspiration and was as wet and as cold as if I had been dragged out of a winter's river.

Another drop fell with a thud like a stone. I would have hidden my head under the bedclothes but I dared not stir. As each drop fell on the bed the interval came quicker until there was a scarlet patch on the white quilt that grew and grew and grew. I felt that the evil stain would come through the coverings, hot and wet, to my clenched hands which were just beneath, but I was unable to move them. My sight was now almost gone. There was nothing but a red haze filling the room, a beating sound in my ears and the drop recurring like the ticking of some awful clock.

I must have become unconscious for I cannot remember

the nurse entering the room. When I realized once more where I was I found that the bedclothes had been changed. There was still the round red mark on the ceiling but it was now dry.

As soon as I could speak I asked, 'Is she dead?' The nurse answered 'No.' 'Will she live?' 'Yes, I hope she will, but it has been a fearful business. The operation lasted two and a quarter hours, and when the great blood vessel gave way they thought it was all over.' 'Was she frightened?' I asked. 'No; she walked into the room, erect and smiling, and said in a jesting voice, "I hope I have not kept you waiting, gentlemen, as I know you cannot begin without me".'

In a week I returned home cured. My 'nerves' were gone. It was absurd to say that I could not walk in the street when that brave woman had walked, smiling, into that place of gags and steel. When I thought of the trouble I had made about going to the play I recalled what had passed in that upper room. I began to think less of my 'case' when I thought of hers.

The doctor was extremely pleased with my recovery; while his belief in the efficacy of the rest cure became unbounded. I did not trouble to tell him that I owed my recovery not to his tiresome physic and ridiculous massage but to that red patch on the ceiling.

The lady of the upper room got well. Through the instrumentality of the nurse I was able to catch sight of her when she was taking her first walk abroad after the operation. I expected to see a goddess. I saw only a plain little woman with gentle eyes and a very white face. I knew that those eyes had peered into eternity.

Some years have now passed by, but still whenever I falter the recollection of that face makes me strong.

TWO WOMEN

In the course of his experience the medical man acquires probably a more intimate knowledge of human nature than is attained by most. He gains an undistorted insight into character. He witnesses the display of elemental passions and emotions. He sees his subject, as it were, unclothed and in the state of a primitive being. There is no camouflage of feeling, no assumption of a part, no finesse. There is merely a man or a woman faced by simple, rudimentary conditions. He notes how they act under strain and stress, under the threat of danger or when menaced by death. He observes their behaviour both during suffering and after relief from pain, the manner in which they bear losses and alarms and how they express the consciousness of joy. These are the common emotional experiences of life, common alike to the caveman and the man of the twentieth century. Among the matters of interest in this purview is the comparative bearing of men and of women when subject to the hand of the surgeon. As to which of the two makes the better patient is a question that cannot be answered in a word. Speaking generally women bear pain better than men. They endure a long illness better, both physically and morally. They are more patient and submissive, less defiant of fate and, I think I may add, more logical. There are exceptions, of course, but then there are exceptions in all things.

Perhaps what the critic of gold calls the 'acid test' is provided by the test of an operation. Here is something very definite to be faced. A man is usually credited with more courage than a woman. This is no doubt a just estimate in situations of panic and violence where less is expected of a woman; but in the cold, deliberate presence of an operation she stands out well.

A display of courage in a man is instinctive, a feature of his upbringing, a matter of tradition. With women is associated a rather attractive element of timidity. It is considered to be a not indecorous attribute of her sex. It is apt to be exaggerated and to become often somewhat of a pose. A woman may be terrified at a mouse in her bedroom and yet will view the entrance into that room of two white-clad inquisitors – the anæsthetist and the surgeon – with composure. A woman will frankly allow, under certain conditions, that she is 'frightened to death'; the man will not permit himself that expression, although he is none the less alarmed. A woman seldom displays bravado; a man often does. To sum up the matter – a woman before the tribunal of the operating theatre is, in my experience, as courageous as a man, although she may show less resolve in concealing her emotions.

In the determination to live, which plays no little part in the success of a grave operation, a woman is, I think, the more resolute. Her powers of endurance are often amazing. Life may hang by a thread, but to that thread she will cling as if it were a straining rope. I recall the case of a lady who had undergone an operation of unusual duration and severity. She was a small, fragile woman, pale and delicate-looking. The blow she had received would have felled a giant. I stood by her bedside some hours after the operation. She was a mere grey shadow of a woman in whom the signs of life seemed to be growing fainter and fainter. The heat of the body was maintained by artificial means. She was still pulseless and her breathing but a succession of low signs. She evidently read anxiety and alarm in the faces of those around her, for, by a movement of her lips, she indicated that she wished to speak to me. I bent down and heard in the faintest whisper the words, 'I am *not* going to die.' She did not die; yet her recovery was a thing incredible. Although twenty-eight years have elapsed since that memorable occasion, I am happy to say that she is still alive and well.

There are other traits in women that the surgeon comes upon which, if not actually peculiar to their sex, are at least displayed by them in the highest degree of perfection. Two of these characteristics – or it may be that the two are one – are illustrated by the incidents which follow.

The first episode may appear to be trivial, although an eminent novelist to whom I told the story thought otherwise and included it, much modified, in one of his books.

The subject was a woman nearing forty. She was plain to look at, commonplace and totally uninteresting. Her husband was of the same pattern and type, a type that embraces the majority of the people in these islands. He was engaged in some humdrum business in the city of London. His means were small and his life as monotonous as a downpour of rain. The couple lived in a small red-brick house in the suburbs. The house was one of twenty in a row. The twenty were all exactly alike. Each was marked by a pathetic pretence to be 'a place in the country'; each was occupied by a family of a uniform and wearying respectability. These houses were like a row of chubby inmates from an institution, all wearing white cotton gloves and all dressed alike in their best.

The street in which the houses stood was called 'The Avenue,' and the house occupied by the couple in question was named 'The Limes.' It was difficult to imagine that anything of real interest could ever occur in 'The Avenue.' It was impossible to associate that decorous road with a murder or even a burglary, much less with an elopement. The only event that had disturbed its peace for long was an occasion when the husband of one of the respected residents had returned home at night in a state of noisy intoxication. For months afterwards the dwellers in 'The Avenue', as they passed that house, looked at it askance. It may be said, in brief, that all the villas were 'genteel' and that all those who lived in them were 'worthy.'

The plain lady of whom I am speaking had no children. She had been happy in a stagnant, unambitious way. Everything went well with her and her household, until one horrifying day when it was discovered that she had developed a malignant tumour of the breast. The growth was operated upon by a competent surgeon, and for a while the spectre was banished. The event, of course, greatly troubled her; but it caused even more anxiety to her husband. The two were very deeply attached. Having few outside interests or diversions, their pleasure in life was bound up with themselves and their small home.

The husband was a nervous and imaginative man. He brooded over the calamity that had befallen his cherished mate. He was haunted by the dread that the horrid thing would come back again. When he was busy at his office he forgot it, and when he was at home and with a wife who seemed in such beaming health it left his mind. In his leisure moments, however, in his journeyings to London and back and in sleepless hours of the night, the terror would come upon him again. It followed him like a shadow.

Time passed; the overhanging cloud became less black and a hope arose that it would fade away altogether. This, however, was not to be. The patient began to be aware of changes at the site of the operation. Unpleasant nodules appeared. They grew and grew and every day looked angrier and more vicious. She had little doubt that 'it' – the awful unmentionable thing – had come back. She dared not tell her husband. He was happy again; the look of anxiety had left his face and everything was as it had been. To save him from distress she kept the dread secret and, although the loathsome thing was gnawing at her vitals, she smiled and maintained her wonted cheerfulness when he and she were together.

She kept the secret too long. In time she began to look ill, to become pallid and feeble and very thin. She struggled on and laughed and joked as in the old days. Her husband was soon aware that something was amiss. Although he dared not express the thought, a presentiment arose in his mind that the thing of terror was coming back. He suggested that she should see her surgeon again, but she pooh-poohed the idea. 'Why should a healthy woman see a surgeon?' At last her husband, gravely alarmed, insisted, and she did as he wished.

The surgeon, of course, saw the position at a glance. The disease had returned, and during the long weeks of concealment had made such progress that any operation or indeed

63

any curative measure was entirely out of the question. Should he tell her? If he told her what would be gained thereby? Nothing could be done to hinder the progress of the malady. To tell her would be to plunge her and her husband into the direst distress. The worry that would be occasioned could only do her harm. Her days were numbered; why not make what remained of her life as free from unhappiness as possible? It was sheer cruelty to tell her. Influenced by these humane arguments he assured her it was all right, patted her on the back and told her to run away home.

For a while both she and her husband were content. She was ready to believe that she had deceived herself and regretted the anxiety she had occasioned; but the unfortunate man did not remain long at ease. His wife was getting weaker and weaker. He wondered why. The surgeon said she was all right; she herself maintained that she was well, but why was she changing so quickly? The doubt and the uncertainty troubled both of them; so it was resolved that a second opinion should be obtained, with the result that she came to see me in London.

A mere glimpse was enough to reveal the condition of affairs. The case was absolutely hopeless as her surgeon, in a letter, had already told me. I was wondering how I should put the matter to her but she made the decision herself. She begged me to tell her the absolute truth. She was not afraid to hear it. She had plans to make. She had already more than a suspicion in her mind and for every reason she must know, honestly and openly, the real state of affairs. I felt that matters were too far gone to justify any further concealment. I told her. She asked if any treatment was possible. I was obliged to answer 'No.' She asked if she would live six months and again I was compelled to answer 'No.'

What happened when she left my house I learned later. It was on a Saturday morning in June that she came to see me. For her husband Saturday was a half-holiday and a day that he looked forward to with eager anticipation. So anxious was he as to my verdict that he had not gone to his business on this particular day. He had not the courage to accompany his wife to London and, indeed, she had begged him not to be present at the consultation. He had seen his wife into the train and spent the rest of the morning wandering listlessly about, traversing every street, road and lane in the neighbourhood in a condition of misery and apprehension.

He knew by what train she would return, but he had not the courage to meet it. He would know the verdict as she stepped out of the carriage and as he caught a glimpse of her face. The platform would be crowded with City friends of his, and whatever the news – good or bad – he felt that he would be unable to control himself.

He resolved to wait for her at the top of 'The Avenue,' a quiet and secluded road. He could not, however, stand still. He continued to roam about aimlessly. He tried to distract his thoughts. He counted the railings on one side of a street, assuring himself that if the last railing proved to be an even number his wife would be all right. It proved to be uneven. He jingled the coins in his pocket and decided that if the first coin he drew out came up 'Heads,' it would be a sign that his wife was well. It came up 'Heads.' Once he found that he had wandered some way from 'The Avenue' and was seized by the panic that he would not get back there in time. He ran back all the way to find, when he drew up, breathless, that he had still twenty-five minutes to wait.

He thought the train would never arrive. It seemed hours and hours late. He looked at his watch a dozen times. At last he heard the train rumble in and pull up at the station. The moment had come. He paced the road to and fro like a caged beast. He opened his coat the better to breathe. He took off his hat to wipe his streaming forehead. He watched the corner at which she would appear. She came suddenly in sight. He saw that she was skipping along, that she was waving her hand and that her face was beaming with smiles. As she approached she called out, 'It is all right!'

He rushed to her, she told me, with a yell, threw his arms round her and hugged her until she thought she would have fainted. On the way to the house he almost danced round her. He waved his hat to everybody he saw and, on entering the house, shook the astonished maid-servant so violently by the hand that she thought he was mad.

That afternoon he enjoyed himself as he had never done before. The cloud was removed, his world was a blaze of sunshine again, his wife was saved. She took him to the golf links and went round with him as he played, although she was so weak she could hardly crawl along. His game was a series of ridiculous antics. He used the handle of his club on the tee, did his putting with a driver and finished up by giving the caddie half a sovereign. In the evening his wife hurriedly invited a few of his choicest friends to supper. It was such a supper as never was known in 'The Avenue' either before or since. He laughed and joked, was generally uproarious, and finished by proposing the health of his wife in a rapturous speech. It was the day of his life.

Next morning she told him the truth.

I asked her why she had not told him at once. She replied, 'It was his half-holiday and I wished to give him just one more happy day.'

The second episode belongs to the days of my youth when I was a house-surgeon. The affair was known in the hospital as 'The Lamp Murder Case.' It concerned a family of three – husband, wife and grown-up daughter. They lived in an ill-smelling slum in the most abject quarter of Whitechapel. The conditions under which this family existed were very evil, although not exceptional in the dark places of any town.

The husband was just a drunken loafer, vicious and brutal, and in his most fitting place when he was lying in the filth of the gutter. He had probably never done a day's work in his life. He lived on the earnings of his wife and daughter. They were seamstresses and those were the doleful days of 'The Song of the Shirt.' As the girl was delicate most of the work fell upon the mother. This wretched woman toiled day by day, from year's end to year's end, to keep this unholy family together. She had neither rest nor relaxation, never a gleam of joy nor a respite from unhappiness. The money gained by fifteen hours' continuous work with her needle might vanish in one uproarious drinking bout. Her husband beat her and kicked her as the fancy pleased him. He did not disable her, since he must have money for drink and she alone could provide it. She could work just as well with a black eye and a bruised body as without those marks of her lord's pleasure.

As she had to work late at night she kept a lamp for her table. One evening the sodden brute, as he staggered into the room, said that he also must have a lamp, must have a lamp of his own. What he wanted it for did not matter. He would have it. He was, as a rule, too muddled to read even if he had ever learnt to read. Possibly he wanted the lamp to curse by. Anyhow, if she did not get him a lamp tomorrow he would 'give her hell,' and the poor woman had already seen enough of hell. Next day she bought a lamp, lit it and placed it on the table with some hope no doubt in her heart that it would please him and bring a ray of peace.

He came home at night not only drunk but quarrelsome. The two lamps were shining together on the table. The room was quite bright and, indeed, almost cheerful; but the spectacle drove him to fury. He cursed the shrinking, tired woman. He cursed the room. He cursed the lamp. It was not the kind of lamp he wanted. It was not so good as her lamp and it was like her meanness to get it. As she stood up to show him how nice a lamp it really was he hit her in the face with such violence that he knocked her into a corner of the room. She was wedged in and unable to rise. He then took up his lamp and, with a yell of profanity, threw it at her as she lay on the ground. At once her apron and cotton dress were ablaze and, as she lay there burning and screaming for mercy, he hurled the other lamp at her.

The place was now lit only by the horrible, dancing flames that rose from the burning woman. The daughter was hiding in terror in the adjoining room. The partition which separated it from her mother's was so thin that she had heard everything that passed. She rushed in and endeavoured to quench the flames; but streams of burning oil were trickling all over the floor, while the saturated clothes on her mother's body flared like a wick. Her father was rolling about, laughing. He might have been a demon out of the Pit. Neighbours

67

poured in and, by means of snatched-up fragments of carpet, bits of sacking and odd clothes, the fire was smothered; but it was too late.

There followed a period of commotion. A crowd gathered in the dingy lane with faces upturned to the window from the broken panes of which smoke was escaping. People pressed up the stair, now thick with the smell of paraffin and of burning flesh. The room, utterly wrecked, was in darkness, but by the light of an unsteady candle stuck in a bottle the body of the woman, moaning with pain, was dragged out. An improvised stretcher was obtained and on it the poor seamstress, wrapped up in a dirty quilt, was marched off to the hospital, followed by a mob. The police had appeared early on the scene and, acting on the evidence of the daughter, had arrested the now terrified drunkard.

When the woman reached the hospital she was still alive but in acute suffering. She was taken into the female accident ward and placed on a bed in a corner by the door. The hour was very late and the ward had been long closed down for the night. It was almost in darkness. The gas jets were lowered and the little light they shed fell upon the white figures of alarmed patients sitting up in bed to watch this sudden company with something dreadful on a stretcher.

A screen was drawn round the burnt woman's bed, and in this little enclosure, full of shadow, a strange and moving spectacle came to pass. The miserable patient was burned to death. Her clothes were reduced to a dark, adhesive crust. In the layers of cinder that marked the front of her dress I noticed two needles that had evidently been stuck there when she ceased her work. Her face was hideously disfigured, the eyes closed, the lips swollen and bladder-like and the cheeks charred in patches to a shiny brown. All her hair was burnt off and was represented by a little greasy ash on the pillow, her eyebrows were streaks of black, while her eyelashes were marked by a line of charcoal at the edge of the lids. She might have been burnt at the stake at Smithfield

As she was sinking it was necessary that her dying depositions should be taken. For this purpose a magistrate was summoned. With him came two policemen, supporting between them the shaking form of the now partly-sobered husband. The scene was one of the most memorable I have witnessed. I can still see the darkened ward, the whispering patients sitting bolt upright in their nightdresses, the darker corner behind the screen, lit only by the light of a hand lamp, the motionless figure, the tray of dressings no longer needed, the half-emptied feeding-cup. I can recall too the ward cat, rudely disturbed, stalking away with a leisurely air of cynical unconcern.

The patient's face was in shadow, the nurse and I stood on one side of the bed, the magistrate was seated on the other. At the foot of the bed were the two policemen and the prisoner. The man – who was in the full light of the lamp – was a disgustful object. He could barely stand; his knees shook under him; his hair was wild; his eyes blood-shot; his face bloated and bestial. From time to time he blubbered hysterically, rocking to and fro. Whenever he looked at his wife he blubbered and seemed in a daze until a tug at his arm by the policeman woke him up.

The magistrate called upon me to inform the woman that she was dying. I did so. She nodded. The magistrate then said to her – having warned her of the import of her evidence – 'Tell me how this happened.' She replied, as clearly as her swollen lips would allow, 'It was a pure accident.'

These were the last words she uttered, for she soon became unconscious and in a little while was dead. She died with a lie on her lips to save the life of the brute who had murdered her, who had burned her alive. She had lied and yet her words expressed a dominating truth. They expressed her faithfulness to the man who had called her wife, her forgiveness for his deeds of fiendish cruelty and a mercy so magnificent as to be almost divine.

A SEA LOVER

The man I would tell about was a mining engineer some forty and odd years of age. Most of his active life had been spent in Africa whence he had returned home to England with some gnawing illness and with the shadow of death upon him. He was tall and gaunt. The tropical sun had tanned his face an unwholesome brown, while the fever-laden wind of the swamp had blanched the colour from his hair. He was a tired-looking man who gave one the idea that he had been long sleepless. He was taciturn, for he had lived much alone and, but for a sister, had no relatives and few friends. For many years he had wandered to and fro surveying and prospecting, and when he turned to look back upon the trail of his life there was little to see but the ever-stretching track, the file of black porters, the solitary camp.

The one thing that struck me most about him was his love of the sea. If he was ill, he said, it must be by the sea. It was a boyish love evidently which had never died out of his heart. It seemed to be his sole fondness and the only thing of which he spoke tenderly.

He was born, I found, at Salcombe, in Devonshire. At that place, as many know, the sea rushes in between two headlands and, pouring over rocky terraces and around sandy bays, flows by the little town and thence away up the estuary. At the last it creeps tamely among meadows and cornfields to the tottering quay at the foot of Kingsbridge.

On the estuary he had spent his early days, and here he and a boy after his own heart had made gracious acquaintance with the sea. When school was done the boys were ever busy among the creeks, playing at smugglers or at treasure seekers so long as the light lasted. Or they hung about the wharf, among the boats and the picturesque litter of the sea, where they recalled in ineffable colours the tales of pirates and the

70

Spanish Main which they had read by the winter fire. The reality of the visions was made keener when they strutted about the deck of the poor semi-domestic coaling brig which leaned wearily against the harbour side or climbed over the bulwarks of the old schooner, which had been wrecked on the beach before they were born, with all the dash of buccaneers.

In their hearts they were both resolved to 'follow the sea' but fate turned their footsteps elsewhere, for one became a mining engineer in the colonies and the other a clerk in a stockbroker's office in London.

In spite of years of uncongenial work and of circumstances which took them far beyond the paradise of tides and salt winds the two boys, as men, ever kept green the memory of the romance-abounding sea. He who was to be a clerk became a pale-faced man who wore spectacles and whose back was bent from much stooping over books. I can think of him at his desk in the City on some day in June, gazing through a dingy window at a palisade of walls and roofs. The clerk's pen is still, for the light on the chimney-pots has changed to a flood of sun upon the Devon cliffs, and the noise of the streets to the sound of waves tumbling among rocks or bubbling over pebbles. There are sea-gulls in the air, while far away a grey barque is blown along before the freshening breeze and the only roofs in view belong to the white cottages about the beach. Then comes the ring of a telephone bell and the dream vanishes.

So with the man whose life was cast in unkindly lands. He would recall times when the heat in the camp was stifling, when the heartless plain shimmered as if it burnt, when water was scarce and what there was of it was warm, while the torment of insects was beyond bearing. At such times he would wonder how the tide stood in the estuary at home. Was the flood swirling up from the Channel, bringing with its clear eddies the smell of the ocean as it hurried in and out among the piles of the old pier? Or was it the time of the ebb when stretches of damp sand come out at the foot of cliffs and when ridges of rock, dripping with cool weed, emerge once

71

more into the sun? What a moment for a swim! Yet here on the veldt there was but half a pint of water in his can and a land stretching before him that was scorched to cracking, dusty and shadowless.

It was in connexion with his illness that I came across him. His trouble was obscure, but after much consideration it was decided that an operation, although a forlorn hope, should be attempted. If the disease proved to be benign there was prospect of a cure; if a cancer was discovered the outlook was hopeless.

He settled that he would have the operation performed at the seaside, at a town on the south coast, within easy reach of London. Rooms were secured for him in a house on the cliffs. From the windows stretched a fine prospect of the Channel, while from them also could be seen the little harbour of the place.

The surgeon and his assistant came down from London and I with them. The room in which the operation was to be performed was hard and unsympathetic. It had been cleared of all its accustomed furniture. On the bare floor a white sheet had been placed, and in the middle of this square stood the operation table like a machine of torture. Beyond the small bed the patient was to occupy and the tables set out for the instruments the room was empty. Two nurses were busy with the preparations for the operation and were gossiping genially in whispers. There was a large bow-window in the room of the type much favoured at seaside resorts. The window was stripped of its curtains so that the sunlight poured in upon the uncovered floor. It was a cloudless morning in July.

The hard-worked surgeon from London had a passion for sailing and had come with the hope that he might spend some hours on the sea after his work was done. His assistant and I were to go with him.

When all the preparations for the operation were completed the patient walked into the room erect and unconcerned. He stepped to the table and, mounting it jauntily, sat on it bolt upright and gazed out earnestly at the sea. Following his eyes I could see that in the harbour the men were already hoisting the mainsail of the little yawl in which we were to sail.

The patient still sat up rigidly, and for so long that the surgeon placed a hand upon his shoulder to motion him to lie down. But he kept fixedly gazing out to sea. Minutes elapsed and yet he moved not. The surgeon, with some expression of anxiety, once more motioned him to lie down, but still he kept his look seawards. At last the rigid muscles relaxed, and as he let his head drop upon the pillow he said, 'I have seen the last of it – the last of the sea – you can do what you like with me now.' He had, indeed, taken, as he thought, farewell of his old love, of the sea of his boyhood and of many happy memories. The eyes of the patient closed upon the sight of the English Channel radiant in the sun, and as the mask of the anæsthetist was placed over his face he muttered, 'I have said good-bye.'

The trouble revealed by the surgeon proved to be cancer, and when, some few days after the operation, the weary man was told the nature of his malady he said, with a smile, he would take no more trouble to live. In fourteen days he died.

Every day his bed was brought close to the window so that the sun could fall upon him, so that his eyes could rest upon the stretch of water and the sound of waves could fall upon his tired ears.

The friend of his boyhood, the clerk, came down from London to see him. They had very little to say to one another when they met. After the simplest greeting was over the sick man turned his face towards the sea and for long he and his old companion gazed at the blue Channel in silence. There was no need for speech. It was the sea that spoke for them. It was evident that they were both back again at Salcombe, at some beloved creek, and that they were boys once more playing by the sea. The sick man's hand moved across the coverlet to search for the hand of his friend, and when the fingers met they closed in a grip of gratitude for the most gracious memory of their lives.

The failing man's last sight of the sea was one evening at

sundown when the tide was swinging away to the west. His look lingered upon the fading waves until the night set in. Then the blind of the window was drawn down.

Next morning at sunrise it was not drawn up, for the lover of the sea was dead.

A CASE OF 'HEART FAILURE'

What a strange company they are, these old patients who crowd into the surgeon's memory after a lifetime of busy practice! There they stand, a confused, impersonal assembly, so illusive and indistinct as to be little more than shadows. Behind them is a dim background of the past – a long building with many windows that I recognize as my old hospital, a consulting room with familiar furniture, an operating theatre, certain indefinite sick-rooms as well as a ward in which are marshalled a double row of beds with blue and white coverlets.

Turning over the pages of old case books, as one would idle with the sheets of an inventory, some of these long departed folk appear clearly enough, both as to their faces and the details of their histories; but the majority are mere ghosts with neither remembered names nor features, neither age nor sex. They are just fragments of anatomy, the last visible portions of figures that are fading out of sight. Here, among the crowd, are the cheeks of a pretty girl encircled by white bandages and the visage of a toothless old man with only one ear. I can recollect nothing but their looks. They belong to people I have known, somewhere and somehow, in the consulting room or the ward. Here a light falls upon 'that knee,' 'that curious skull,' 'that puzzling growth.' Here is a much distorted back, bare and pitiable, surmounted by coils of beautiful brown hair. If the lady turned round I should probably not recognize her face; but I remember the back and the coils of hair.

This is a gathering, indeed, not of people, but of 'cases' recalled by portions of their bodies. The collection is not unlike a medley of fragments of stained glass with isolated pieces of the human figure painted upon them, or it may be comparable to a faded fresco in a cloister, where the portions that survive, although complete in themselves, fail to recall the story they once have told.

It is curious, when so much is indefinite, how vividly certain trivial items stand forth as the sole remains of a once complete personality. All I can recall of one lady – elderly but sane – was the fact that she always received me, during a long illness, sitting up in bed with a large hat on her head trimmed with red poppies. She also wore a veil, which she had to lift in order that I might see her tongue. She was further distinguished by a rose pinned to her nightdress, but I recall with relief that she did not wear gloves.

Of one jolly boy the only particular that survives in my mind is a hare's foot which was found under his pillow when he was awaiting an operation. It had been a talisman to coax him to sleep in his baby days, when his small hand would close upon it as the world faded. His old 'nanny' had brought it to the nursing home, and had placed it secretly under his pillow, knowing that he would search for it in the unhappy daze of awakening from chloroform. He wept with shame when it was discovered, but I am sure it was put back again under the pillow, although he called his 'nanny' 'a silly old thing.'

Then, again, there was the whistling girl. She was about sixteen, and had recently learnt whistling from a brother. Her operation had been serious, but she was evidently determined to face it sturdily and never to give way. She expressed herself by whistling, and the expression was even more realistic than speech. Thus as I came upstairs the tone of her whistling was defiant and was intended to show that she was not the least afraid. During the dressing of the wound the whistling was subdued and uncertain, a rippling accompaniment that conveyed content when she was not hurt, but that was interrupted by a staccato 'whoo' when there was a dart of pain. As soon as my visit was over the music became debonair and triumphant, so that I often left the room to the tune of Mendelssohn's 'Wedding March.'

On the other hand, among the phantoms of the case book are some who are remembered with a completeness which

76

appears never to have grown dim. The figures are entire, while the inscription that records their story is as clear as it was when it was written.

In the company of these well remembered people is the lady whose story is here set forth. More than thirty years have passed since I saw her, and yet I can recall her features almost as well as if I had met her yesterday, can note again her little tricks of manner and the very words she uttered in our brief conferences. She was a woman of about twenty-eight, small and fragile; and very pretty. Her face was oval, her complexion exquisite, while her grey-blue eyes had in them the look of solemn wonder so often seen in the eyes of a child. Her hair came down low on either side of her face, and was so arranged as to remind me of the face of some solemn lady in an old Italian picture. Her mouth was small and sensitive, but determined, and she kept her lips a little apart when listening. She was quiet and self-possessed, while her movements and her speech were slow, as if she were weary.

She was shown into my room at an hour when I did not, as a rule, receive patients. She came without appointment and without any letter of introduction from her doctor. She said that she had no doctor, that she came from a remote place in the north of England, that she had an idea what was the matter with her, and that she wanted me to carry out the necessary operation. On investigation I found that she had an internal growth which would soon imperil her life. I explained to her that an operation would be dangerous and possibly uncertain, but that if it proved successful her cure would be complete. She said she would have the operation carried out at once, and asked me to direct her to a nursing home. She displayed neither anxiety nor reasonable interest. Her mind was made up. As to any danger to her life, the point was not worth discussing.

She had informed me that she was married, but had no children. I inquired as to her parents, but she replied that she was an orphan. I told her that I must write fully both to her doctor and to her husband. She replied, as before, that she had no doctor, and that it seemed a pity to worry a strange medical man with details about a patient who was not under his care. As to her husband, she asked if I had told her all and if there would be anything in my letter to him that I had not communicated to her. I said that she knew the utmost I had to tell. 'In that case,' she replied, 'a note from you is unnecessary.' I said, 'Of course, your husband will come up to London?' To which she remarked, 'I cannot see the need. He has his own affairs to attend to. Why should any fuss be made? The operation concerns no one but myself.'

I asked her then what relative or friend would look after her during the operation. She said, 'No one. I have no relatives I care about; and as to friends, I do not propose to make my operation a subject for gossip.' I explained to her that under such circumstances no surgeon would undertake the operation. It was a hazardous measure, and it was essential that she should have someone near her during a period of such anxiety. She finally agreed to ask an elderly lady – a remote connexion of hers – to be with her during her stay in the nursing home.

Still, there was some mystery about the lady that I could not fathom, something evidently that I did not know. There was a suggestion of recklessness and even of desperation in her attitude that it was difficult to account for. As she sat in the chair by the side of my desk, with her hands folded in her lap and her very dainty feet crossed in front of her, her appearance of indifference was so pronounced that no onlooker would imagine that the purport of our converse was a matter of life and death. One little movement of hers during our unemotional talk was recalled to my mind some days later. She now and then put her hand to her neck to finger a brooch in the collar of her dress. It was a simple gold brooch, but she appeared to derive some comfort, or it may be some confidence, from the mere touching of it.

The operation was effected without untoward incident of any kind. It was entirely successful. The wound healed by what is known as 'first intention,' there was no rise of temperature and no surgical complication. But the condition of the patient caused an uneasiness that deepened day by day.

She became restless and apathetic and at the same time very silent, answering questions only in monosyllables. She resisted no detail of treatment, but accepted everything with a lethargic complacency impossible to overcome.

That, however, was not all. She appeared to be possessed by an indefinite anxiety which was partly expressed by an intense attitude of expectation. She was expecting a letter, looking out for it day after day and hour after hour. She listened to the door and to any sound on the stair as an imprisoned dog might listen for the steps of its master. This terrible vigil began on the second or third day after the operation. When I made my visit about that time she asked me if I had given orders that she was to have no letters. I assured her I had not done so and that she should have every letter the moment it arrived. But no letter came.

Whenever I made my appearance her first question was, 'Did you see a letter for me in the hall?' I could only answer 'No.' Then she would press me with other inquiries: 'How often does the postman come? Is he not sometimes late? Has there been any accident on the railway? Do letters get occasionally lost in the post?' and so on interminably. If anyone came into the room there was always a look of expectation on her face, an eager searching for a letter in the hand or on a tray. If a knock was heard at the front door, she at once inquired if it was the postman, and very usually asked me to go to the top of the stair to ascertain.

The sisters, the nurses and the patient's friend could tell me nothing. No letter of any kind arrived. The poor, tormented creature's yearning for a letter had become a possession. I inquired if she had written any letters herself. The sister said that, as far as was known, she had written but one, and that was on the eve of her operation. Although she should have been in bed at the time, she insisted on going out for the purpose of posting the letter herself.

She rapidly became weaker, more restless, more harassed by despair. She was unable to sleep without drugs and took scarcely any food. Feeble and failing as she was, her anxiety about the coming of a letter never abated. I asked a physician versed in nervous disorders to see her, but he had little to propose. She was evidently dying – but of what?

She was now a pitiable spectacle, emaciated and hollow-eyed, with a spot of red on her cheek, an ever-wrinkled brow and ever-muttering lips. I can see to this day the profile of her lamentable features against the white background of the pillow. Pinned to the pillow was the brooch that I had noticed at her neck when I saw her in my consulting room. She would never allow it to be removed, but gave no reason for her insistence. I have seen her hand now and then move up to touch it, just as she had done during our first interview.

I was with her when she died. As I entered the room there was still the same expectant glance at the door. Her lips, dry and brown, appeared to be shaping the question, 'A letter for me?' There was no need to answer 'No.' At the very last – with a display of strength that amazed me – she turned over with her face to the wall as if she wished to be alone; then, in a voice louder than I had known her to be capable of for days, she cried out, 'Oh, Frank! Frank!' and in a moment later she was dead.

Her death was certified, with unconscious accuracy, as due to 'heart failure.'

Here was a mystery, and with it a realization of how little we knew of this lady who had died because she wished to die. I was aware that her husband's christian name was William, but beyond that I knew practically nothing of him. The sister of the nursing home had both written and telegraphed to the husband, but no reply had been received. It was afterwards ascertained that he was away at the time and that the house was shut up.

I was determined to find out the meaning of the tragedy, but it was some months before I was possessed of the whole of the story. The poor lady's marriage had been unhappy. Her husband had neglected her, and they were completely estranged. She formed a friendship with a man of middle age who lived near by. This is he whose christian name was Frank and who was, I imagine, the giver of the brooch. The friendship grew into something more emotional. She

80

became, indeed, desperately attached to him, and he to her. Their intimacy was soon so conspicuous as to lead to gossip in the neighbourhood, while the state of the two lovers themselves was one of blank despair. She looked to him as Pompillia looked to Caponsacchi. He was her saviour, her 'soldier saint, the lover of her life.' To him she could repeat Pompillia's words: 'You are ordained to call and I to come.'

It became evident in time that the only course the two could adopt was to run away together. She, on her part, counted no cost and would have followed him blindly to the world's end. He, on the other hand, hesitated. He did count the cost and found it crushing. His means were small.

His future depended on himself. An elopement would involve ruin, poverty and squalor as well as, in time, a fretful awakening from a glorious dream.

He did the only thing possible. He told her that they must part, that he must give her up, that he must not see her again, that he must not even write to her. It was a wise and, indeed, inevitable decision; but to her it seemed to foretell the end of her life. He kept the compact, but she had not the strength to accept it. It was something that was impossible. She endeavoured to get in touch with him again and again, and in many ways, but without success. Hard as it was, he had kept to his resolve.

Then came the episode of the operation. Now, she thought, if she wrote to him to say that she was in London and alone and that she was about to undergo an operation that might cause her death, he must come to see her or he must at least reply to her letter. She felt assured that she would hear from him at last, for, after all that had passed between them, he could not deny her one little word of comfort in this tragic moment.

She wrote to him on the eve of her operation. The rest of the story I have told.

A RESTLESS NIGHT

It was in Rajputana, in the cold weather, that we came upon the dâk bungalow. I was proceeding south from a native state where I had met an officer in the Indian Medical Service. He was starting on a medical tour of inspection, and for the first stage of the journey we travelled together. He was glad to have a member of his own profession to talk to.

Towards the end of the day we halted at this dâk bungalow. It was situated in a poor waste which was possessed of two features only – dried earth and cactus bushes. So elemental was the landscape that it might have been a part of the primeval world before the green things came into being. The cactus, bloated, misshaped and scarred by great age, looked like some antediluvian growth which had preceded the familiar plants with leaves. If a saurian had been in sight browsing on this ancient scrub the monster would have been in keeping. Some way distant across the plain was a native village, simple enough to be a settlement of neolithic men. Although it was but a splash of brown amidst the faded green it conveyed the assurance that there were still men on the earth.

The bungalow was simple as a packing-case. It showed no pretence at decoration, while there was in its making not a timber nor a trowel of plaster which could have been dispensed with. In the centre of the miserly place was a common room with a veranda in front and a faintly-suggested kitchen at the back. Leading out of the common room, on either side, was a bedroom, and the establishment was complete. The central room was provided with one meal-stained table and two dissolute-looking chairs of the kind found in a servant's attic. The walls were bare save for certain glutinous splashes where insects had been squashed by the slipper of some tormented guest. The place smelt of grease and paraffin, toned by a faint suggestion of that unclean aromatic odour which clings to Indian dwellings. The bedrooms were alike – square chambers with cement floors, plain as an empty water-tank. An inventory of their respective contents was completed by the following items – one low bedstead void of bedding, one chair, one table with traces of varnish in places and one looking-glass in a state of desquamation. To these may be added one window and two doors. One door led into the common room, the other into a cemented bathroom containing a battered tin bath, skinned even of its paint.

We each of us had an Indian servant or bearer who, with mechanical melancholy, made the toilet table pretentious by placing upon it the entire contents of our respective dressing bags.

After dinner, of a sort, we sat on the penitential chairs and smoked, leaning our elbows on the table for our greater comfort. The doctor was eloquent upon his medical experiences in the district, upon his conflicts with pessimistic patients and his struggles with fanaticism and ignorance. The average sick man, he told me, had more confidence in a dried frog suspended from the neck in a bag than in the whole British Pharmacopœa. Most of his narratives have passed out of my memory, but one incident I had reason to remember.

It concerned a native from the adjacent village who was working as a stone-mason and whose eye was pierced by a minute splinter of stone. As a result the eye became inflamed and sightless, save that the man retained in the damaged organ an appreciation of light. As bearing upon the case and its sequel I must explain the circumstances of 'sympathetic ophthalmia.' When an eye is damaged as this was, and inflammation ensues, it is not uncommon for the mischief to spread to the sound globe and destroy that also. In order to prevent such a catastrophe it is necessary to remove the injured and useless eye as promptly as possible. That was the uniform practice in my time. The operation in question was urged upon the native in order to prevent sympathetic ophthalmia in the sound eye, but he declined it, preferring to consult a magician who lived a day's journey from the village.

The consultation took place and the man returned to the local dispensary; for although he still had good vision in the sound eye it was beginning to trouble him.

The surgeon considered that the operation was now probably too late; but he yet urged it upon the ground that there was some prospect of success, while, on the other hand, failure could make the patient's condition no more desperate. The man, persuaded against his will, at last consented, and the useless eyeball was removed. Unfortunately the operation *was* too late; the sound eye became involved beyond recovery and the miserable native found himself totally blind. He ignorantly ascribed his loss of sight to the operation.

Before my friend left the station the man was brought into his room for the last time, and when it was explained to him that he was in the doctor's presence he threw his arms aloft and, shrieking aloud, cursed the man of healing with a vehemence which should have brought down fire from heaven. He called upon every deity in the Indian mythology to pour torments upon this maimer of men, to blast his home and annihilate his family root and branch. He blackened the sky with curses because the darkness which engulfed him prevented him from tearing out with his nails the eyes of this murderous Englishman. Foaming and screaming, and almost voiceless from the violence of his speech, he was led away to stumble about his village, where for weeks he rent the air with his awful imprecations. Whether the poor man was now alive or dead the doctor could not say, for he had heard no more of him.

In due course we agreed that the time had come to go to bed. The doctor said that he always occupied the right-hand bedroom when he came to the bungalow, but as it was found that my servant had deposited my bedding and effects in this particular sepulchre, he retired to the chamber across the hall.

I did not look forward to a night in this so called 'Rest House.' The bedroom was as comfortless as a prison cell and as desolate as the one sound room in a ruin. There was some comfort in contemplating the familiar articles displayed on the dressing-table, yet they looked curiously out of place.

I locked the door leading to the common room, but found that the door to the bathroom had no lock; while there was merely a bolt to the outer door that led from the bathroom into the open. This bolt I shot, but left the intermediate door ajar, feeling that I should like to assure myself from time to time that the far room was empty. There was one small paraffin lamp provided, but the glass shade of it had been broken, so that it was only when the wick was very low that it would burn without smoking. By the glimmer of this malodorous flame I undressed and, blowing it out, got into bed.

The place was as black as a pit, as stifling and as silent. I lay awake a long time, for the stillness was oppressive. I found myself listening to it. It seemed to be made up of some faint, far-off sounds of mysterious import of which I imagined I could catch the rhythm. It was possible to believe that these half-imagined pulsations were produced by the rush of the earth through space, and that the stillness of the night made them audible.

I went to sleep in time and slept – as I afterwards discovered – for some hours, when I was aroused by a noise in the room. I was wide awake in an instant, with my head raised off the pillow, listening rigidly for the sound that I must have heard in my sleep. The place was in solid darkness. I felt that there was something alive in the room, something that moved.

At last the sound came again. It was the pattering of the feet of some animal. The creature was coming towards the bed. I could hear others moving along the floor, always from the bathroom, until the place seemed to be alive with invisible creatures. Such is the effect of imagination that I conceived these unknown animals to be about the size of retrievers. I wondered if their heads would reach the level of the couch, until I was relieved to hear that many were now running about under the bed. I resolved to shout at them but fancied that the noise of my own voice would be as unpleasant to hear as the voice of another and unknown human being in the room.

I noticed now a faint odour of musk, and was glad to think that these pattering feet belonged to musk-rats, and that these animals must have entered through the drain hole I had observed in the outer wall of the bathroom. I dislike rats, and especially rats in a bedroom. This prejudice was not made less when I felt that some of them were climbing up on to the bed. I was certain I could hear one crawling over my clothes which lay on the chair by the bedside. I was certain that others were searching about on the dressing-table, and recognized – or thought I did – the clatter of a shoe-horn that lay there. I recalled stories in which men had been attacked by hordes of rats, and I wondered when they would attack me, for, by this time, the whole room seemed to be full of rats, and I could picture legions swarming in from the plain outside in a long snake-like column.

In a while I was sure that a rat was on the pillow close to my head. My hair seemed to be flicked by the whiskers of one of these fœtid brutes. This was more than I could tolerate, so I sprang up in bed and shouted. There was a general scuttle for the far door; but it was some time before I ventured to pass my hand over the pillow to assure myself that a rat was not still there.

I had a mind to get out of bed and light the lamp; but to do this seemed to be like taking a step into a black pit. I lay down again. For a while all was quiet. Then came once more the pattering of feet from the direction of the bathroom, the sickly odour of musk and a conviction that at least a hundred rats were pouring into the room. They crept up to the bed and ran about beneath it with increasing boldness. I was meditating another shout when there came a sound in the room that made every vein in my body tingle. It arose from under the bed, a hollow scraping sound which I felt sure was due to the movement of a human being. I thought it was caused by the scraping of a belt buckle on the cement floor, the belt being worn by a man who was crawling on his stomach. I disliked this sound more than the rats.

At this moment, to add to my discomfort, I felt a rat crawling across my bare foot, a beast with small, cold paws and hot fur. I kicked it off so that it fell with a thud on the floor. I shouted again and, driven to desperation, jumped out of bed. I half expected to tread on a mass of rats, but felt the hard floor instead. I went to the dressing-table and struck a light. The place was empty, but I could not see under the bed. The match went out and in the blackness I expected some fresh surprise to develop. I managed to strike another match and to light the lamp.

I placed it on the floor and looked under the bed. What I saw there I took at first to be a piece of a human skull. I got a stick and touched it. It seemed lighter than a dried bone. I dragged it out into the room. It was a cake of unleavened bread, much used by the natives – dried up into a large curled chip. The rats had been dragging this away and had so produced the scraping sound which I had exaggerated into something sinister.

Having convinced myself that the room was empty I blocked up the drain-hole in the outer wall by placing the bath in front of it and, feeling secure from any further disturbance, returned to bed, leaving the lamp alight on the table.

For a long time I kept awake, watching every now and then the bathroom door to satisfy myself that I had succeeded in keeping the beastly animals out. During this vigil I fell asleep and then at once embarked upon a dream, the vividness and reality of which were certainly remarkable.

The most convincing feature was this. The dream, without a break, continued the happenings of the night. The scene was this identical bedroom at this identical moment. The dream, as it were, took up the story from the moment that I lost it. Owing to my close scrutiny every detail of the vile chamber had already become as clearly impressed upon my brain as if it had been fixed by a photographic plate. I had not – in my dream – fallen asleep again, but was still wide awake and still keeping a watch over the bathroom door for the incoming of the rats.

The bathroom door was just ajar, but the very faint glimmer of the lamp did not enable me to penetrate the darkness that filled it. I kept my eye fixed on the entry when, in a moment, to my horror, the door began to open. The sight was terrifying in the extreme. My heart was thumping to such a degree that I thought its beats must be audible. I felt a deadly sinking in my stomach, while the skin of my back and neck seemed to be wrinkling and to be dragged up as might be a shirt a man is drawing over his head. There is no panic like the panic felt in a dream.

A brown hand appeared on the edge of the door. It was almost a relief to see that it was a human hand. The door was then opened to its utmost. Out of the dark there crept a middle-aged man, a native, lean and sinewy, without a vestige of clothing on his body. His skin shone in the uncertain light, and it was evident that his body, from head to foot, was smeared with oil. The most noticeable point about the man was that he was blind. His eyelids were closed, but the sockets of his eyes were sunken as are those of a corpse. With his left hand he felt for the wall, while in his right hand he carried a small stonemason's pick. His face was expressionless. This was the most terrible thing about it, for his face was as the face of the dead. He crept into the room as Death himself might creep into the chamber of the dying.

I realized at once in my dream that this was the native about whom my friend had been speaking before we had retired for the night. This man had heard of the doctor's arrival, would know my room as the one he usually occupied, and had now come there to murder him.

I was so fascinated by the sight of this unhuman creature moving towards me that I could not stir a muscle. I was raised up in bed, and was leaning on one elbow like an image on a tomb. I was so filled with the sense of a final calamity that I felt I had ceased to breathe. There were, indeed, such a clutching at my throat and such a bursting at my heart that the act of breathing seemed wellnigh impossible. Had I been awake I should, without doubt, have shouted at the uncanny intruder and attacked him, but in the dream I was unable to

88

stir, and the longer I remained motionless the more impossible did it appear that I could move. My limbs might have been turned into stone.

The figure crept on, feeling his way by the wall. There was a sense of an oncoming, irresistible fate. Every time that a horrible bare foot was lifted, advanced and brought to the ground I felt that I was one step nearer to the end. The figure seemed to grow larger as it approached me. The hand, with outstretched fingers, that groped its way along the wall was like a claw. I could hear the breathing of the creature, the breath being drawn in between the closed teeth. I could see the muscles of the arm that held the pick contract and relax. There was now in the air the loathsome smell of the unclean native mixed with the odour of oil.

One more step and he was so near that I could see the faint light glimmer on his teeth and could notice that they were dry. The outstretched, claw-like hand that felt its way along the wall was now nearly over my head. In another moment that awful pick would crash into my skull or plunge into my neck. I bowed my head instinctively so that I should not see the blow coming, and at the same time I thought it would be less terrible if the iron were driven into my back rather than into my head or face.

The evil creature was now close to the bed. The extended arm was clawing along the wall above my pillow, for I had now shrunken as low as I could. With my head bent I could now see nothing of the man but his wizened thigh, upon which the muscles rose and fell. A bony knee-cap was advanced slowly, and then I saw a shadow move on the floor. This I felt was the shadow of the arm with the pick raised to strike.

I was mesmerized as would be a rabbit in a corner within a foot of a snake. Suddenly the lamp flame gave a little crackle. The sound, breaking the silence, was intensified into an explosion. It seemed to call me to my senses. With one maddened half-conscious effort I rolled gently off the bed, away from the pursuer, and slipped, between the couch and the wall, on to the floor.

I made little noise in doing this, for my body was uncovered, the bed was very low, and the space between it and the wall so narrow that I was let slowly down to the ground. To the blind man I may merely have turned in bed.

As I lay there on the floor I could see the two sinewy feet close to the couch and could hear the awful hand moving stealthily over the very pillow. I next knew that he was bending over the couch to find what was between the bed and the wall. Turning my head, I saw a shadowy hand descend on the far side of the bed, the fingers extended as if feeling the air. In a moment he would reach me. His hand moved to and fro like the head of a cobra, while I felt that with a touch of his tentacle-like fingers I should die. The climax of the dream was reached.

I was now well under the bed. In a paroxysm of despair I seized the two skinny ankles and jerked them towards me, at the same moment lifting the frail bed bodily with my back so that it turned over on its side away from the wall. The wretch's feet being suddenly drawn away from him, he fell heavily backwards upon the bare floor, his head striking the stone with a hollow sound. The edge of the bedstead lay across him. The feet, which I still held, were nerveless, and he made no movement to withdraw them. I crept back clear of the bed and, jumping upright against the wall, bolted through the bathroom and out into the plain. I had a glimpse of the man as I went by. He was motionless and his mouth hung open.

I ran some way from the bungalow before I stopped. I was like a man saved from the scaffold as the very axe was about to drop. There was a gentle air blowing, cool and kindly. Above was a sky of stars, while in the east the faint light of the dawn was appearing behind the Indian village.

For a moment or two I watched the door leading from the bathroom, expecting to see the man with the pick creep out, but the anticipation of the sight was so dread that I turned away and walked to the other side of the bungalow. Here my greatest joy was merely to breathe, for I seemed to have been for hours in a suffocating pit.

The relief did not last for long. I was seized with another panic. Had I killed the man? I felt compelled to return to the abhorred room and learn the worst. I approached it with trembling. So curious are the details of a dream that I found – as I expected – the bolt on the outer door wrenched off and hanging by a nail. I stepped into the disgusting place, full of anxiety as to what further horror I had to endure. The little lamp was still alight. The bedstead was on its edge as I left it, but the man was gone. There was a small patch of blood where his head had struck the floor, but that was the sole relic of the tragedy.

I awoke feeling exhausted, alarmed and very cold. I looked at once at the floor for the patch of blood, and, seeing nothing, realized, to my extreme relief, that I had been merely dreaming. It was almost impossible to believe that the events of the latter part of the night, after the departure of the rats, had not been real. At breakfast I retailed to my companion the very vivid and dramatic nightmare in which I had taken part. At the end he expressed regret for the mistake the servants had made in allotting us our rooms overnight, but I am not sure that that regret was perfectly sincere.

IN ARTICULO MORTIS

The recent work on 'Death and its Mystery',* by Camille Flammarion, the eminent astronomer, cannot fail to be of supreme interest. The second volume of the series, entitled 'At the Moment of Death', will more especially appeal to medical men, and it is with this volume and with the reminiscences it has aroused that I am at present concerned.

About the act or process of dying there is no mystery. The pathologist can explain precisely how death comes to pass, while the physiologist can describe the exact physical and chemical processes that ensue when a living thing ceases to live. Furthermore, he can demonstrate how the material of the body is finally resolved into the elements from which it was formed.

The mystery begins in the moment of death, and that mystery has engaged the thoughts and imaginations of men since the dawn of human existence. It was probably the first problem that presented itself to the inquisitive and ingenious mind, and it may be that it will be the last to occupy it. Beyond the barrier of death is 'the undiscovered country' where a kindly light falls upon Elysian Fields or happy hunting grounds, or fills with splendour the streets of an eternal city. To some, on the other hand, there is no such country but only an impenetrable void, a blank, a mere ceasing to be. Certain who read these works of the learned astronomer may perhaps feel that he has thrown light upon the great mystery. Others may affirm that he leaves that mystery still unillumined and wholly unsolved, while others again may think that he makes the mystery still more mysterious and more complex.

M. Flammarion deals with the manifestations of the dying, with agencies set in action by the dying, and with events

*Fisher Unwin, London, 1922.

92

which attend upon the moment of death. He affirms that in addition to the physical body there is an astral body or 'psychic element' which is 'imponderable and gifted with special, intrinsic faculties, capable of functioning apart from the physical organism, and of manifesting itself at a distance'.

This leads to the theory of bilocation where the actual body (at the point of death) may be in one place and the astral body in another. It is this power of bilocation which explains the phantasms and apparitions of which the book gives many detailed records. These apparitions may be objective – that is to say, may be visible to several people at the same time – or they may be subjective or capable of being perceived only by the subject or seer. 'These apparitions,' the author states, 'are projections emanating from the soul of the dying.' They are astral bodies detached for the moment from the physical body of which they are part. 'It is,' the author continues, 'at the hour of death that transmissions of images and of sensations are most frequent' (p. 108).

These phantasms appear, either in dreams or in broad daylight, to the friends of dying persons. They may announce in words, 'I am dying,' or 'I am dead.' They may merely appear with signs upon their faces of alarm or of impending dissolution. They may appear as bodies lying dead upon a couch or in a coffin. They may predict the hour of their death, but more usually their appearance coincides with the exact moment at which their physical bodies ceased to exist.

M. Flammarion gives numerous instances of these apparitions seen under such varying circumstances as have been named. In certain examples the phantom appears to have substance and to be capable of making its presence actually felt. Thus in one case the subject saw the apparition of her sister who was dying in a place far away, and at the same time 'felt a hand brush lightly against the sheets'. The subject, when questioned, said: 'No, no, it wasn't a dream! I heard her steps; they made the floor creak. I'm sure of it; I wasn't dreaming; she came; I saw her' (p. 345).

It may be further noted that persons who announce their

deaths to others by visions or by spoken words may at the time of such warning be in perfect health. Moreover, the apparition may announce to the dreamer the exact date of the speaker's own death many days in advance. In one such instance a man – then in sound health – appeared to a friend in a dream on August 2 and informed him that he (the subject of the apparition) would die on August 15. The event happened as foretold. An instance which involved an interval of years is recorded by Robert Browning the poet. Seven years after his wife's death she appeared in a dream to her sister, Miss Arabel Barrett. Miss Barrett asked the apparition, 'When will the day come on which we shall be reunited?' The dead woman answered, 'My dear, in five years.' Five years, lacking a month, after this vision, Miss Barrett died of heart disease.

In messages or warnings from the dying M. Flammarion affirms that telepathy (or the transmission of thought to a distance) plays an important part. More than this, he says: 'It is beyond doubt that at the moment of death a subtle shock, unknown in its nature, at times affects those at a distance who are connected with the dying person in some way. This connexion is not always that of sympathy.' The method in which telepathy acts is explained by the author in the following words: 'It is admitted that a kind of radiation emanates from the dying person's brain, from his spirit, still in his body, and is dispersed into space in ether waves – successive, spherical waves, like those of sound in the atmosphere. When this wave, this emanation, this effluvium, comes into contact with a brain attuned to receive it, as in the case of a wireless-telegraph apparatus, the brain comprehends it – feels, hears, sees' (p. 284).

The manifestations produced by these passages between the living and those who are on the point of death are very varied. They may take the form of warnings, predictions or notifications of death. They may be conveyed vast distances and are usually received at the very moment at which the body from which they emanate ceases to be. Warnings or announcements may be conveyed by voices or by visions of various kinds. The voices may be recognized as those of the dying, or the actual death scene, 'visioned from a distance', may be presented complete in every detail. Some of the manifestations may take a physical form, such as knockings upon doors and windows, the sound of footsteps or of gliding feet, the moving of articles of furniture, the falling of portraits from the wall, the opening of doors, the passage of a gust of wind.

Many of the phenomena appear to me to be hardly worthy of being recorded. As illustrations I may quote the movement of a hat on a hat peg used by the deceased, the violent shaking of an iron fender to announce a daughter's death, the fact that about the time of a relative's decease a table became 'split completely along its whole length', while on another like occasion a gas jet went out in a room in which a party was sitting, playing cards.

The following circumstance will not commend itself to the reasonable as one that was dependent upon a supernatural agency. 'My grandmother,' a student writes, 'died in 1913. At the hour of her death the clock which hung in her room stopped, and no one could make it go again. Some years afterwards her son died, and the very day of his death the clock again began to go without anyone having touched it.' 'It is strange,' comments M. Flammarion, 'that the spirit of someone dying or dead should be able to stop a clock or start it again.' Assuredly it is more than strange. The same comment might apply to the following testimony provided by a gardener in Lunéville. 'A friend, when one day cleaning vegetables, seated in a chair, was struck on the knee by a turnip which was on the ground, and heard at the same instant two cries: "Mother! Mother!" That same day her son, a soldier, was dying in our colony of Guiana; she did not hear of his death until very much later.'

M. Flammarion's work is probably the most orderly, temperate and exact that has appeared on the subject of death from the point of view of the spiritualist. It has been the work of many years and its conclusions are based upon hundreds of reports, letters and declarations collected by the writer. To many readers the book will, no doubt, be convincing and inspiring, while possibly to a larger number of people the author's position will appear to be untenable, and much of the evidence upon which his conclusions are based to be either incredible or impossible. With those who may hold this latter opinion I am entirely in accord.

Many of the so-called manifestations, such as the spirit visitants, the visions and the voices, can be as fitly claimed to be illusions and hallucinations as affirmed to be due to the action of the psychic element or astral body. The tricks of the senses are innumerable. The imagination, stimulated and intensified, can effect strange things in sensitive subjects; while, on the other hand, the powers of self-deception are almost beyond belief, as the experience of any physician will attest. Belief in the supernatural and the miraculous has a fascination for many minds, and especially for minds of not too stable an order. Such persons seem to prefer a transcendental explanation to one that is commonplace. Apparitions are not apt to appear to those who are healthy both in body and in mind. Dreams, it will be admitted by all, are more often due to indigestion than to a supernatural or a spiritual agency. Voices are heard and non-existing things are seen by those whose minds are deranged, and it must be allowed that not a few of the men and women upon whose evidence M. Flammarion depends exhibit a degree of emotional excitement or exaltation which borders on the abnormal.

I think, moreover, it would not be unjust to suggest that certain of the narratives are exaggerated and that an element of invention is possible and, indeed, probable in many of them. There is an impression also that some of the circumstances detailed have been misinterpreted or mis-applied or have been modified by events which have followed later and to which they have been adapted as an afterthought. Above all I am reluctant to believe that the dying, in the solemn and supreme moment of passing away from the earth, can be occupied by the trivialities – and, indeed, I would say by the paltry tricks – which are accredited to their action in this book.

It is only fair to point out that the volume now discussed is written by an eminent man of science who has been trained all his life in methods of precision, in the judicial examination of reported facts and in the close scrutiny of evidence. Further it may be said that the terms 'incredible' and 'impossible' would have been applied a few years ago to any account of the telephone or of wireless telegraphy, while the same expressions would assuredly be employed by a medical man when told, not so long since, that there was a ray capable of making a human body so transparent as to render visible not only the bones but the details of their internal construction.

In common with others who have been for many years on the staff of a large hospital, I have seen much of death and have heard even more from those who have been in attendance on the dying. In this experience of a lifetime I have never met with a single circumstance which would confirm or support the propositions advanced by M. Flammarion. This is obviously no argument. It is merely a record of negative experience. The only two events, within my personal knowledge, which bear even remotely upon the present subject are the following.

I was, as a youth, on a walking tour in the south of England with a cousin. We put up one night at a certain inn. In the morning my companion came down to breakfast much excited and perturbed. He declared that his father was dead, that in a vivid dream he had seen him stretched out dead upon the couch in his familiar bedroom at home. He had awakened suddenly and noted that the hour was 2 A.M. That his father had expired at that moment he was assured, so assured that he proposed to return home at once, since his mother was alone. Inasmuch as the journey would have occupied a whole day, I suggested that, before starting, he should telegraph and seek news of his father. With great reluctance he consented to this course and the telegram was dispatched. A reply was received in due course. It was from the father himself expressing surprise at the inquiry and stating that he was never better in his life. Nothing, it transpired, had disturbed the father's rest at 2 A.M. on this particular night. Nothing untoward happened. My uncle lived for many years, and finally died one afternoon, and not, therefore, at 2 A.M.

The other incident is associated with an actual death and with a strange announcement, but the announcement is not to be explained by any of the theories propounded by M. Flammarion. The facts are these. I was on a steamship which was making a passage along that coast known in old days as the Spanish Main. We put in at Colon, and remained there for about a day and a half. I took advantage of this break in the voyage to cross the Isthmus by train to Panama. The names of those who were travelling by the train had been telegraphed to that city, which will explain how it came about that on reaching the station I was accosted by one of the medical officers of the famous American hospital of the place. He begged me to see with him a patient under his care. The sick man was an Englishman who was travelling for pleasure, who was quite alone and who had been taken ill shortly after his arrival on the Pacific. He was the only Englishman, he said, on that side of the Isthmus.

I found the gentleman in a private ward. He was a stranger to me, was very gravely ill, but still perfectly conscious. I had nothing fresh to suggest in the way of treatment. The case was obviously hopeless, and we agreed that his life could not be extended beyond a few days and certainly not for a week. It was a satisfaction to feel that the patient was as well cared for as if he had been in his own home in England. I returned to Colon. Travelling with me was a retired general of the Indian Army. He had remained at Colon during my absence. I told him my experience. He did not know the patient even by name, but was much distressed at the thought of a fellow-countryman dying alone in this somewhat remote part of the world. This idea, I noticed, impressed him greatly.

Two days after my return from Panama we were on the high seas, having touched at no port since leaving Colon. On the third day after my visit to the hospital the general made a curious communication to me. The hour for lunch on the steamer was 12.15. My friend, as he sat down to the table, said abruptly, 'Your patient at Panama is dead. He has just died. He died at 12 o'clock.' I naturally asked how he had acquired this knowledge, since we had called nowhere, there was no wireless installation on the ship, and we had received no message from any passing vessel. Apart from all this was the question of time, for the death, he maintained, had only just occurred. He replied, 'I cannot say. I was not even thinking of the poor man. I only know that as the ship's bell was striking twelve I was suddenly aware that he had, at that moment, died.' The general, I may say, was a man of sturdy common sense who had no belief in the supernatural, nor in emanations from the dying, nor in warnings, nor in what he called generally 'all that nonsense'. Telepathy – in which also he did not believe – was out of the question, since he and the dead man were entirely unknown to one another. My friend was merely aware that the news had reached him. It was useless for me to say that I did not think the patient could have died so soon, for the general remained unmoved. He only knew that the man was dead whether I expected the event or whether I did not.

When we reached Trinidad I proposed to go ashore to ascertain if any news had arrived of the death at Panama. The general said it was waste of time. The man was dead, and had died at noon. Nevertheless, I landed and found that a telegram had appeared in which the death of this lonely gentleman was noted as having taken place on the day I have named. The hour of his death was not mentioned, but on my return to England I was shown by his relatives the actual cablegram which had conveyed to them the news. It stated that he had died at Panama on that particular day at twelve o'clock noon. No coincidence could have been more precise.

The general, to whom the event was as mysterious as it was unique in his experience, ventured one comment. He said that during his long residence in India he had heard rumours of the transmission of news from natives in one part of India to natives in another, which reports – if true – could not be explained by the feats of runners nor by any system of signalling, since the distances traversed were often hundreds of miles. We were both aware of the rumour, current at the time, that the news of the defeat at Colenso was known in a certain Indian bazaar a few hours after the guns had ceased firing. This, we agreed, was assuredly an example of loose babble – started by a native who hoped to hear of the failure of the British – and that this gossip had become, by repetition, converted into a prophecy after the occurrence.

For my own part I must regard the Panama incident as nothing but a remarkable coincidence of thought and event. My friend was inclined to regard it as an example of the sudden transmission of news of the kind suggested by his Indian experience. Why he of all people should have been the recipient of the message was beyond his speculation, since he had no more concern with the happenings at Panama than had the captain of the ship, to whom I had also spoken of the occurrence.

A further subject of some interest, suggested by M. Flammarion's work, may be touched upon. In the contemplation of the mystery of death it may be reasonable to conjecture that at the moment of dying, or in the first moment after death, the great secret would be, in whole or in part, revealed. There are those who believe that after death there is merely the void of non-existence, the impenetrable and eternal night of nothingness. Others conceive the spirit of the dead as wandering, somewhere and somehow, beyond the limits of the world. It is this belief which has induced many a mother, after the death of her child, to leave the cottage door open and to put a light in the window with some hope that the wandering feet might find a way home. Others, again, hold to the conviction that those who die pass at once into a new state of existence, the conditions of which vary according to the faith of the believer.

In the face of the great mystery it would be thought that those who have returned to life after having been, for an appreciable time, apparently dead might have gained some insight into the unknown that lies beyond. Cases of such recovery are not uncommon, and not a few must have come within the experience of most medical men of large practice. I have watched certain of such cases with much interest. Among them the most pronounced example of apparent lifelessness was afforded by the following occasion.

A middle-aged man, in good general health, was brought into the theatre of the London Hospital to undergo an operation of a moderate degree of severity. The administration of an anæsthetic was commenced, but long before the moment for operating arrived the man collapsed and appeared to be dead. His pulse had stopped, or at least no pulse could be detected, the heartbeat could not be felt, he had ceased to breathe, all traces of sensation had vanished, and his countenance was the countenance of the dead. Artificial respiration was at once employed, injections of various kinds were given, electricity was made extended use of, while the heat of the body was maintained by hot bottles liberally disposed.

The man remained without evidence of life for a period so long that it seemed to be impossible that he could be other than dead. In the intense anxiety that prevailed, and in the excitement aroused, I have no doubt that this period of time was exaggerated and that seconds might have been counted as minutes; but it represented, in my own experience, the longest stretch of time during which a patient has remained apparently without life. Feeble indications of respiration returned and a flutter at the wrist could again be felt, but it was long before the man was well enough to be moved back to the ward, the operation having been, of course, abandoned.

I determined to watch the recovery of consciousness in this instance, for here was a man who had been so far dead that, for a period almost incredible to believe, he had been without the signs and evidences of life. If life be indicated by certain manifestations, he had ceased to live. He was, without question, apparently dead. It seemed to me that this man must have penetrated so far into the Valley of the Shadow of Death that he should have seen something of what was beyond, some part, at least, of the way, some trace of a path, some sight of a country. The door that separates life from death was in his case surely opening. Had he no glimpse as it stood ajar?

He became conscious very slowly. He looked at me, but I evidently conveyed no meaning to his mind. He seemed gradually to take in the details of the ward, and at last his eye fell upon the nurse. He recognized her, and after some little time said, with a smile, 'Nurse, you never told me what you heard at the music hall last night.' I questioned him later as to any experience he may have had while in the operating theatre. He replied that, except for the first unpleasantness of breathing chloroform, he remembered nothing. He had dreamed nothing.

At a recent meeting (1922) of the British Medical Association at Glasgow Sir William MacEwen reports an even more remarkable case of a man who was brought into the hospital as 'dead'. He had ceased to breathe before admission. An operation upon the brain was performed without the use of an anaesthetic of any kind. During the procedure artificial respiration was maintained. The man recovered consciousness and, looking round with amazement at the operating theatre and the strange gathering of surgeons, dressers and nurses, broke his death-like silence by exclaiming, 'What's all this fuss about?' It is evident from cases such as these that no light upon the mystery is likely to be shed by the testimony of those who have even advanced so far as to reach at least the borderland of the 'undiscovered country'.

I might conclude this fragment with some comment on the Fear of Death. The dread of death is an instinct common to all humanity. Its counterpart is the instinct of self-preservation, the resolve to live. It is not concerned with the question of physical pain or distress, but is the fear of extinction, a dread of leaving the world, with its loves, its friendships and its cherished individual affairs, with perhaps hopes unrealized and projects incomplete. It is a dread of which the young know little. To them life is eternal. The adventure is before them. Death and old age are as far away as the blue haze of the horizon. It is about middle age that the realization dawns upon men that life does not last for ever and that things must come to an end. As the past grows vaster and more distant and the future lessens to a mere span, the dread of death diminishes, so that in extreme old age it may be actually welcomed.

Quite apart from this natural and instinctive attitude of mind there is with many a poignant fear of death itself, of the actual act of dying and of the terror and suffering that may be thereby involved. This fear is ill-founded. The last moments of life are more distressing to witness than to endure. What is termed 'the agony of death' concerns the watcher by the bedside rather than the being who is the subject of pity. A last illness may be long, wearisome and painful, but the closing moments of it are, as a rule, free from suffering. There may appear to be a terrible struggle at the end, but of this struggle the subject is unconscious. It is the onlooker who bears the misery of it. To the subject there is merely a moment:

> 'When something like a white wave of the sea
> Breaks o'er the brain and buries us in sleep.'

Death is often sudden, may often come during sleep, or may approach so gradually as to be almost unperceived. Those who resent the drawbacks of old age may take some consolation from the fact that the longer a man lives the easier he dies.

A medical friend of mine had among his patients a very old couple who, having a few remaining interests in the world, had taken up the study and arrangement of their health as a kind of hobby or diversion. To them the subject was like a game of 'Patience', and was treated in somewhat the same way. They had made an arrangement with the doctor that he should look in and see them every morning. He would find them, in the winter, in a cosy, old-fashioned room, sitting round the fire in two spacious arm-chairs which were precisely alike and were precisely placed, one on the right hand and one on the left. The old lady, with a bright ribbon in her lace cap and a shawl around her shoulders, would generally have some knitting on her knees, while the old gentleman, in

103

a black biretta, would be fumbling with a newspaper and a pair of horn spectacles.

The doctor's conversation every morning was, of necessity, monotonous. He would listen to accounts of the food consumed, of the medicine taken and of the quantity of sleep secured, just as he would listen to the details of a game of 'Patience'. Now and then there would be some startling 'move', some such adventure as a walk to the garden gate or the bold act of sitting for an hour at the open window. After having received this report he would compliment the lady on her knitting and on the singing of her canary and would discuss with the gentleman such items of news as he had read in the paper.

On one morning visit he found them as usual. The wife was asleep, with her spectacles still in place and her hands folded over her knitting. The canary was full of song. The midday beef tea was warming on the hob. The old gentleman, having dealt with his health, became very heated on the subject of certain grievances, such as the noise of the church bells and the unseemly sounds which issued from the village inn. He characterized these and like disturbances of the peace as 'outrages which were a disgrace to the country'. After he had made his denunciation he said he felt better.

'Your wife, I see, is asleep,' said the doctor. 'Yes,' replied the old man; 'she has been asleep, I am glad to say, for quite two hours, because the poor dear had a bad night last night.' The doctor crossed the room to look at the old lady. She was dead, and had, indeed, been dead for two hours. Such may be the last moments of the very old.

Quite commonly the actual instant of death is preceded, for hours or days, by total unconsciousness. In other instances a state of semi-consciousness may exist up to almost the last moment of life. It is a dreamy condition, free of all anxiety, a state of twilight when the familiar landscape of the world is becoming very indistinct. In this penumbra friends are recognized, automatic acts are performed, and remarks are uttered which show, or seem to show, both purpose and reason. It is, however, so hazy a mental mood that could the individual return to life again no recollection of the period would, I think, survive. It is a condition not only free from uneasiness and from any suspicion of alarm, but is one suggestive even of content.

I was with a friend of mine – a solicitor – at the moment of his death. Although pulseless and rapidly sinking, he was conscious, and in the quite happy condition just described. I suggested that I should rearrange his pillows and put him in a more comfortable position. He replied, 'Don't trouble, my dear fellow; a lawyer is comfortable in any position.' After that he never spoke again.

THE IDOL WITH HANDS OF CLAY

The good surgeon is born, not made. He is a complex product in any case, and often something of a prodigy. His qualities cannot be expressed by diplomas nor appraised by university degrees. It may be possible to ascertain what he knows, but no examination can elicit what he can do. He must know the human body as a forester knows his wood; must know it even better than he, must know the roots and branches of every tree, the source and wanderings of every rivulet, the banks of every alley, the flowers of every glade. As a surgeon, moreover, he must be learned in the moods and troubles of the wood, must know of the wild winds that may rend it, of the savage things that lurk in its secret haunts, of the strangling creepers that may throttle its sturdiest growth, of the rot and mould that may make dust of its very heart. As an operator, moreover, he must be a deft handicraftsman and a master of touch.

He may have all these acquirements and yet be found wanting; just as a man may succeed when shooting at a target, but fail when faced by a charging lion. He may be a clever manipulator and yet be mentally clumsy. He may even be brilliant, but Heaven help the poor soul who has to be operated upon by a brilliant surgeon. Brilliancy is out of place in surgery. It is pleasing in the juggler who plays with knives in the air, but it causes anxiety in an operating theatre.

The surgeon's hands must be delicate, but they must also be strong. He needs a lacemaker's fingers and a seaman's grip. He must have courage, be quick to think and prompt to act, be sure of himself and captain of the venture he commands. The surgeon has often to fight for another's life. I conceive of him then not as a massive Hercules wrestling ponderously with Death for the body of Alcestis, but as a nimble man in doublet and hose who, over a prostrate form, fights Death with a rapier.

These reflections were the outcome of an incident which had set me thinking of the equipment of a surgeon and of what is needed to fit him for his work. The episode concerned a young medical man who had started practice in a humble country town. His student career had been meritorious and indeed distinguished. He had obtained an entrance scholarship at his medical school, had collected many laudatory certificates, had been awarded a gold medal and had become a Fellow of the Royal College of Surgeons. His inclination was towards surgery. He considered surgery to be his *métier*. Although circumstances had condemned him to the drab life of a family doctor in a little town, he persisted that he was, first and foremost, a surgeon, and, indeed, on his door-plate had inverted the usual wording and had described himself as 'surgeon and physician.' In his hospital days he had assisted at many operations, but his opportunities of acting as a principal had been few and insignificant. In a small practice in a small town surgical opportunities are rare. There was in the place a cottage hospital with six beds, but it was mostly occupied by medical cases, by patients with rheumatism or pneumonia, by patients who had to submit to the surgical indignity of being poulticed and of being treated by mere physic. Cases worthy of a Fellow of the Royal College of Surgeons were very few, and even these seldom soared in interest above an abscess or a broken leg.

Just before the young doctor settled down to practise he married. It was a very happy union. The bride was the daughter of a neighbouring farmer. She had spent her life in the country, was more familiar with the ways of fowls and ducks than with the ways of the world, while a sunbonnet became her better than a Paris toque. She was as pretty as the milkmaid of a pastoral picture with her pink-and-white complexion, her laughing eyes and her rippled hair.

Her chief charm was her radiant delight in the mere joy of living. The small world in which she moved was to her always in the sun, and the sun was that of summer. There was no town so pretty as her little town, and no house so perfect as 'the doctor's' in the High Street. 'The doctor's' was a Georgian house with windows of many panes, with a fanlight like a surprised eyebrow over the entry and a self-conscious brass knocker on the door. The house was close to the pavement, from which it was separated by a line of white posts connected by loops of chain. Passers-by could look over the low green wooden blinds into the dining-room and see the table covered with worn magazines, for the room was intended to imitate a High Street waiting-room. They could see also the bright things on the sideboard, the wedding-present biscuit box, the gong hanging from two cow-horns and the cup won at some hospital sports. To the young wife there never was such a house, nor such furniture, nor such ornaments, nor, as she went about with a duster from room to room, could there be a greater joy than that of keeping everything polished and bright.

Her most supreme adoration, however, was for her husband. He was so handsome, so devoted, and so amazingly clever. His learning was beyond the common grasp, and the depths of his knowledge unfathomable. When a friend came in at night to smoke a pipe she would sit silent and open-mouthed, lost in admiration of her husband's dazzling intellect. How glibly he would talk of metabolism and blood-pressure; how marvellously he endowed common things with mystic significance when he discoursed upon the value in calories of a pound of steak, or upon the vitamines that enrich the common bean, or even the more common cabbage. It seemed to her that behind the tiny world she knew there was a mysterious universe with which her well-beloved was as familiar as was she with the contents of her larder.

She was supremely happy and content, while her husband bestowed upon her all the affection of which he was capable. He was naturally vain, but her idolatry made him vainer. She considered him wonderful, and he was beginning to think her estimate had some truth in it. She was so proud of him that she rather wearied her friends by the tale of his achievements. She pressed him to allow her to have his diploma and his more florid certificates framed and hung up in the consulting room, but he had said with chilling superiority that such things 'were not done,' so that she could only console herself by adoring the modesty of men of genius.

One day this happy, ever-busy lady was seized with appendicitis. She had had attacks in her youth, but they had passed away. This attack, although not severe, was graver, and her husband determined, quite wisely, that an operation was necessary. He proposed to ask a well-known surgeon in a neighbouring city to undertake this measure. He told his wife, of course, of his intention, but she would have none of it. 'No,' she said, 'she would not be operated on by stuffy old Mr. Heron.* He was no good. She could not bear him even to touch her. If an operation was necessary no one should do it but her husband. He was so clever, such a surgeon, and so up-to-date. Old Heron was a fossil and behind the times. No! Her clever Jimmy should do it and no one else. She could trust no one else. In his wonderful hands she would be safe, and would be running about again in the garden in no time. What was the use of a fine surgeon if his own wife was denied his precious help!'

The husband made no attempt to resist her wish. He contemplated the ordeal with dread, but was so influenced by her fervid flattery that he concealed from her the fact that the prospect made him faint of heart and that he had even asked himself: 'Can I go through with it?'

He told me afterwards that his miserable vanity decided him. He could not admit that he lacked either courage or competence. He saw, moreover, the prospect of making an impression. The town people would say: 'Here is a surgeon so sure of himself that he carries out a grave operation on his own wife without a tremor.' Then, again, his assistant would be his fellow-practitioner in the town. How impressed he would be by the operator's skill, by his coolness, by the display of the latest type of instrument, and generally by his very advanced methods. It was true that it was the first major

* The name is fictitious.

operation he had ever undertaken, but he no longer hesitated. He must not imperil his wife's faith in him nor fail to realize her conception of his powers. As he said to me more than once, it was his vanity that decided him.

He read up the details of the operation in every available manual he possessed. It seemed to be a simple procedure. Undoubtedly in nine cases out of ten it *is* a simple measure. His small experience, as an onlooker, had been limited to the nine cases. He had never met with the tenth. He hardly believed in it. The operation as he had watched it at the hospital seemed so simple, but he forgot that the work of expert hands does generally appear simple.

The elaborate preparations for the operation – made with anxious fussiness and much clinking of steel – were duly completed. The lady was brought into the room appointed for the operation and placed on the table. She looked very young. Her hair, parted at the back, was arranged in two long plaits, one on either side of her face, as if she were a schoolgirl. She had insisted on a pink bow at the end of each plait, pleading that they were cheerful. She smiled as she saw her husband standing in the room looking very gaunt and solemn in his operating dress – a garb of linen that made him appear half-monk, half-mechanic. She held her hand towards him, but he said he could not take it as his own hand was sterilized. Her smile vanished for a moment at the rebuke, but came back again as she said: 'Now don't look so serious, Jimmy; I am not the least afraid. I know that with you I am safe and that you will make me well, but be sure you are by my side when I awake, for I want to see you as I open my eyes. Wonderful boy!'

The operation was commenced. The young doctor told me that as he cut with his knife into that beautiful white skin and saw the blood well up behind it a lump rose in his throat and he felt that he must give up the venture. His vanity, however, urged him on. His doctor friend was watching him. He must impress him with his coolness and his mastery of the position. He talked of casual things to show that he was quite at ease, but his utterances were artificial and forced.

For a time all went well. He was showing off, he felt, with some effect. But when the depths of the wound were reached a condition of things was found which puzzled him. Structures were confused and matted together, and so obscured as to be unrecognizable. He had read of nothing like this in his books. It was the tenth case. He became uneasy and, indeed, alarmed, as one who had lost his way. He ceased to chatter. He tried to retain his attitude of coolness and command. He must be bold, he kept saying to himself. He made blind efforts to find his course, became wild and finally reckless. Then a terrible thing happened. There was a tear – something gave way – something gushed forth. His heart seemed to stop. He thought he should faint. A cold sweat broke out upon his brow. He ceased to speak. His trembling fingers groped aimlessly in the depths of the wound. His friend asked: 'What has happened?' He replied with a sickly fury: 'Shut up!'

He then tried to repair the damage he had done; took up instrument after instrument and dropped them again until the patient's body was covered with soiled and discarded forceps, knives and clamps. He wiped the sweat from his brow with his hand and left a wide streak of blood across his forehead. His knees shook and he stamped to try to stop them. He cursed the doctor who was helping him, crying out: 'For God's sake do this,' or 'For God's sake don't do that'; sighed like a suffocating man; looked vacantly round the room as if for help; looked appealingly to his wife's masked face for some sign of her tender comfort, but she was more than dumb. Frenzied with despair, he told the nurse to send for Mr. Heron. It was a hopeless mission, since that surgeon – even if at home – could not arrive for hours.

He tried again and again to close the awful rent, but he was now nearly dropping with terror and exhaustion. Then the anæsthetist said in a whisper: 'How much longer will you be? Her pulse is failing. She cannot stand much more.' He felt that he must finish or die. He finished in a way. He closed the wound, and then sank on a stool with his face buried in his blood-stained hands, while the nurse and the doctor applied the necessary dressing.

The patient was carried back to her bedroom, but he dared not follow. The doctor who had helped him crept away without speaking a word. He was left alone in this dreadful room with its hideous reminders of what he had done. He wandered about, looked aimlessly out of the window, but saw nothing, picked up his wife's handkerchief which was lying on the table, crunched it in his hand, and then dropped it on the floor as the red horror of it all flooded his brain. What had he done to her? She! She of all women in the world!

He caught sight of himself in the glass. His face was smeared with blood. He looked inhuman and unrecognizable. It was not himself he saw: it was a murderer with the brand of Cain upon his brow. He looked again at her handkerchief on the ground. It was the last thing her hand had closed upon. It was a piece of her lying amid this scene of unspeakable horror. It was like some ghastly item of evidence in a murder story. He could not touch it. He could not look at it. He covered it with a towel.

In a while he washed his hands and face, put on his coat and walked into the bedroom. The blind was down; the place was almost dark; the atmosphere was laden with the smell of ether. He could see the form of his wife on the bed, but she was so still and seemed so thin. The coverlet appeared so flat, except where the points of her feet raised a little ridge. Her face was as white as marble. Although the room was very silent, he could not hear her breathe. On one side of the bed stood the nurse, and on the other side the anæsthetist. Both were motionless. They said nothing. Indeed, there was nothing to say. They did not even look up when he came in. He touched his wife's hand, but it was cold and he could feel no pulse.

In about two hours Heron, the surgeon, arrived. The young doctor saw him in an adjacent bedroom, gave him an incoherent, spasmodic account of the operation, laid emphasis on unsurmountable difficulties, gabbled something about an accident, tried to excuse himself, maintained that the fault was not his, but that circumstances were against him.

The surgeon's examination of the patient was very brief. He went into the room alone. As he came out he closed the door after him. The husband, numb with terror, was awaiting him in the lobby. The surgeon put his hand on the wretched man's shoulder, shook his head and, without uttering a single word, made his way down the stairs. He nearly stumbled over a couple of shrinking, white-faced maids who had crept up the stairs in the hope of hearing something of their young mistress.

As he passed one said: 'Is she better, doctor?' but he merely shook his head, and without a word walked out into the sunny street where some children were dancing to a barrel-organ.

The husband told me that he could not remember what he did during these portentous hours after the operation. He could not stay in the bedroom. He wandered about the house. He went into his consulting room and pulled out some half-dozen works on surgery with the idea of gaining some comfort or guidance; but he never saw a word on the printed page. He went into the dispensary and looked over the rows of bottles on the shelves to see if he could find anything, any drug, any elixir that would help. He crammed all sorts of medicines into his pocket and took them upstairs, but, as he entered the room, he forgot all about them, and when he found them in his coat a week later he wondered how they had got there. He remembered a pallid maid coming up to him and saying: 'Lunch is ready, sir.' He thought her mad.

He told me that among the horrors that haunted him during these hours of waiting not the least were the flippant and callous thoughts that would force themselves into his mind with fiendish brutality. There was, for example, a scent bottle on his wife's table – a present from her aunt. He found himself wondering why her aunt had given it to her and when, what she had paid for it, and what the aunt would say when she heard her niece was dead. Worse than that, he began composing in his mind an obituary notice for the

113

newspapers. How should he word it? Should he say 'beloved wife,' or 'dearly loved wife,' and should he add all his medical qualifications? It was terrible. Terrible, too, was his constant longing to tell his wife of the trouble he was in and to be comforted by her.

Shortly after the surgeon left the anæsthetist noticed some momentary gleam of consciousness in the patient. The husband hurried in. The end had come. His wife's face was turned towards the window. The nurse lifted the blind a little so that the light fell full upon her. She opened her eyes and at once recognized her husband. She tried to move her hand towards him, but it fell listless on the sheet. A smile – radiant, grateful, adoring – illumined her face, and as he bent over her he heard her whisper: 'Wonderful boy.'

BREAKING THE NEWS

Among the more painful experiences which haunt a doctor's memory are the occasions on which it has been necessary to tell a patient that his malady is fatal and that no measure of cure lies in the hands of man. Rarely indeed has such an announcement to be bluntly made. In the face of misfortune it is merciless to blot out hope. That meagre hope, although it may be but a will-o'-the-wisp, is still a glimmer of light in the gathering gloom. Very often the evil tidings can be conveyed by the lips of a sympathetic friend. Very often the message can be worded in so illusive a manner as to plant merely a germ of doubt in the mind; which germ may slowly and almost painlessly grow into a realization of the truth. I remember being present when Sir William Jenner was enumerating to a friend the qualities he considered to be essential in a medical man. 'He needs,' said the shrewd physician, 'three things. He must be honest, he must be dogmatic and he must be kind.' In imparting his dread message the doctor needs all these qualities, but more especially the last – he must be kind. His kindness will be the more convincing if he can, for the moment, imagine himself in the patient's place and the patient in his.

The mind associates the pronouncing of a verdict and a sentence of death with a court of justice, a solemn judge in his robes, the ministers of the law, the dock, a pallid and almost breathless audience. Such a spectacle, with its elaborate dignity, is impressive enough, but it is hardly less moving when the scene is changed to a plain room, hushed almost to silence and occupied by two persons only, the one who speaks and the one who listens – the latter with bowed head and with knotted hands clenched between his knees.

The manner in which ill-news is received depends upon its gravity, upon the degree to which the announcement is unexpected and upon the emotional bearing of the recipient. There may be an intense outburst of feeling. There may be none. The most pitiable cases are those in which the sentence is received in silence, or when from the trembling lips there merely escapes the words, 'It has come.'

The most vivid displays of feeling that occur to my mind have been exhibited by mothers when the fate of a child is concerned. If her child be threatened a mother may become a tigress. I remember one such instance. I was quietly interviewing a patient in my consulting room when the door suddenly flew open and there burst in – as if blown in by a gust of wind – a gasping, wild-eyed woman with a little girl tucked up under her arm like a puppy. Without a word of introduction she exclaimed in a hoarse whisper, 'He wants to take her foot off.' This sudden, unexplained lady was a total stranger to me. She had no appointment. I knew nothing of her. She might have dropped from the clouds. However, the elements of violence, confusion and terror that she introduced into my placid room were so explosive and disturbing that I begged my patient to excuse me and conducted, or rather impelled, the distraught lady into another room. Incidentally I may remark that she was young and very pretty; but she was evidently quite oblivious of her looks, her complexion, her dress or her many attractions. I had before noticed that when a good-looking woman is unconscious of being good-looking there is a crisis in progress.

The story, which was told me in gasps and at white heat, was as follow. The child was a little girl of about three, almost as pretty as her mother. She was the only child and had developed tuberculous disease in one foot. The mother had taken the little thing to a young surgeon who appears to have let fall some rash remark as to taking the foot off. This was enough for the mother. She would not listen to another syllable. She, whom I came to know later as one of the sweetest and gentlest of women, changed at the moment to a wild animal – a tigress.

Without a word she snatched up the baby and bolted from the house, leaving the child's sock and shoe on the

116

consulting-room floor. She had been given my name as a possible person to consult and had dashed off to my house, carrying the child through the streets with its bare foot and leg dangling in the air. On being admitted she asked which was my room. It was pointed out to her, and without more ado she flung herself in as I have described. The child, I may say, was beaming with delight. This dashing in and out of other people's houses and being carried through the streets without a sock or a shoe on her foot struck her as a delicious and exciting game.

The mother's fury against my surgical colleague was almost inexpressible. If the poor man had suggested cutting off the child's head he could not have done worse. 'How dare he!' she gasped. 'How dare he talk of cutting off her foot! If he had proposed to cut off my foot I should not have minded. It would be nothing. But to cut off her little foot, this beautiful little foot, is a horror beyond words, and then look at the child, how sweet and wonderful she is! What wickedness!' It was a marvellous display of one of the primitive emotions of mankind, a picture, in human guise, of a tigress defending her cub. By a happy good fortune, after many months and after not a few minor operations, the foot got well so that the glare in the eyes of the tigress died away and she remembered again that she was a pretty woman.

It is well known that the abrupt reception of ill-tidings may have a disastrous effect upon the hearer. The medical man is aware that, if he would avoid shock, the announcement of unpleasant facts or of unhappy news must be made slowly and with a tactful caution. In this method of procedure I learnt my lesson very early and in a way that impressed my memory.

I was a house-surgeon and it was Christmas time. In my day each house-surgeon was on what was called 'full duty' for one entire week in the month. During these seven days all accident cases came into his surgeon's wards. He was said to be 'taking in.' On this particular Christmas week I was 'taking in.' Two of my brother house-surgeons had obtained short leave for Christmas and I had undertaken their duties.

It was a busy time; so busy indeed that I had not been to bed for two nights. On the eve of the third night I was waiting for my dressers in the main corridor at the foot of the stair. I was leaning against the wall and, for the first and the last time in my life, I fell asleep standing up. The nap was short, for I was soon awakened, 'rudely awakened' as novelists would put it.

I found myself clutched by a heated and panting woman who, as she clung to me, said in a hollow voice, 'Where have they took him?' The question needed some amplification. I inquired who 'he' was. She replied, 'The bad accident case just took in.' Now the term 'accident' implies, in hospital language, a man ridden over in the street, or fallen from a scaffold, or broken up by a railway collision. I told her I had admitted no such case of accident. In fact the docks and the great works were closed, and men and women were celebrating the birth of Christ by eating too much, by getting drunk and by street rioting, which acts involved only minor casualties. She was, however, convinced he was 'took in.' He was her husband. She gave me his name, but that conveyed nothing, as it was the dresser's business to take names. With a happy inspiration I asked, 'What is he?' 'A butler,' she replied. Now a butler is one of the rarest varieties of mankind ever to be seen in Whitechapel, and it did so happen that I had, a few hours before, admitted an undoubted butler. I told her so, with the effusion of one eager to give useful information. She said, 'What is the matter with him?' I replied cheerily, 'He has cut his throat.'

The effect of this unwise readiness on my part was astonishing. The poor woman, letting go of my coat, collapsed vertically to the floor. She seemed to shut up within herself like a telescope. She just went down like a dress dropping from a peg. When she was as small a heap as was possible in a human being she rolled over on to her head on the ground. A more sudden collapse I have never seen. Had I been fully awake it would never have happened. We placed her on a couch and soon restored her to consciousness.

Her story was simple. She and her husband had met. The two being 'full of supper and distempering draughts' (as

118

Brabantio would say) had had a savage quarrel. At the end he banged out of the house, exclaiming, 'I will put an end to this.' She had bawled after him, 'I hope to God you will.' He had wandered to Whitechapel and, creeping into a stable, had cut his throat there and then. The friend who hastened to inform the wife told her, with a tactfulness I so grievously lacked, that her husband had met with an accident and had been taken to the hospital. This lesson I never forgot and in the future based my method of announcing disaster upon that adopted by the butler's discreet friend.

Although a digression from the present subject I am reminded of the confusion that occasionally took place in the identity of cases. All patients in the hospital who are seriously ill, whether they have been long in the wards or have been only just admitted, are placed on 'the dangerous list' and have their names posted at the gate so that their relatives might be admitted at any time of the day or night.

A man very gravely injured had been taken into the accident ward. He was insensible and his condition such that he was at once put on the dangerous list, or, in the language of the time, was 'gated.' During the course of the evening a youngish woman, dressed obviously in her best, bustled into the ward with an air of importance and with a handkerchief to her lips. She demanded to see the man who had been brought in seriously injured. She was directed by the sister to a bed behind a screen where lay the man, still insensible and with his head and much of his face enveloped in bandages. The woman at once dropped on her knees by the bedside and, throwing her arms about the neck of the unconscious man, wept with extreme profusion and with such demonstrations of grief as are observed at an Oriental funeral. When she had exhausted herself she rose to her feet and, staring at the man on the bed, exclaimed suddenly, 'This is not Jim. This is not my husband. Where is he?'

Now, in the next bed to the one with the screen, and in full view of it, was a staring man sitting bolt upright. He had been admitted with an injury to the knee. This was Jim. He was almost overcome by amazement. He had seen his wife, dressed in her best, enter the ward, clap her hand to her forehead, fall on her knees and throw her arms round the neck of a total stranger and proceed to smother him with kisses. Jim's name had been 'gated' by mistake.

When she came to the bedside of her real husband she was annoyed and hurt, so hurt, indeed, that she dealt with him rudely. She had worked herself up for a really moving theatrical display in the wards, had rehearsed what she should say as she rode along in the omnibus and considered herself rather a heroine or, at least, a lady of intense and beautiful feeling which she had now a chance of showing off. All this was wasted and thrown away. An injured knee, caused by falling over a bucket, was not a subject for fine emotional treatment. She was disgusted with Jim. He had taken her in. 'Bah!' she exclaimed. 'Come in with water on the knee! You might as well have come in with water on the brain! You are a fraud, you are! What do you mean by dragging me all the way here for nothing? You ought to be ashamed of yourself.' With this reproof she sailed out of the room with great dignity – a deeply injured woman.

To return to the original topic. In all my experience the most curious manner in which a painful announcement was received was manifested under the following circumstances. A gentleman brought his daughter to see me – a charming girl of eighteen. He was a widower and she was his only child. A swelling had appeared in the upper part of her arm and was increasing ominously. It became evident on examination that the growth was of the kind known as a sarcoma and that the only measure to save life was an amputation of the limb at the shoulder joint, after, of course, the needful confirmatory exploration had been made.

A more distressing position could hardly be imagined. The girl appeared to be in good health and was certainly in the best of spirits. Her father was absolutely devoted to her. She was his ever-delightful companion and the joy and comfort of his life. Terrible as the situation was it was essential not only that the truth should be told but told at once. Everything depended upon an immediate operation and, therefore, there was not a day to be lost. To break the news seemed for a moment almost impossible. The poor father had no suspicion of the gravity of the case. He imagined that the trouble would probably be dealt with by a course of medicine and a potent liniment. I approached the revelation of the dreadful truth in an obscure manner. I discussed generalities, things that were possible, difficulties that might be, threw out hints, mentioned vague cases, and finally made known to him the bare and ghastly truth with as much gentleness as I could command.

The wretched man listened to my discourse with apparent apathy, as if wondering what all this talk could mean and what it had to do with him. When I had finished he said nothing, but, rising quietly from his chair, walked over to one side of the room and looked at a picture hanging on the wall. He looked at it closely and then, stepping back and with his head on one side, viewed it at a few feet distant. Finally he examined it through his hand screwed up like a tube. While so doing he said, 'That is a nice picture. I rather like it. Who is the artist? Ah! I see his name in the corner. I like the way in which he has treated the clouds, don't you? The foreground too, with those sheep, is very cleverly managed.' Then turning suddenly to me he burst out, 'What were you talking about just now? You said something. What was it? For God's sake say that it is not true! It is not true! It cannot be true!'

A QUESTION OF HATS

I had had a very busy afternoon and had still two appointments to keep. The first of these was in the suburbs, a consultation with a doctor who was a stranger to me. It was a familiar type of house where we met – classic Doric pillars to the portico, a congested hall with hat-pegs made of cow horns, a pea-green vase with a fern in it perched on a bamboo tripod, and a red and perspiring maid-servant. Further, I became acquainted with a dining-room containing bomb-proof, mahogany furniture, and great prints in pairs on the walls, 'War' and 'Peace' on one side, 'Summer' and 'Winter' on the other. Then there was the best bedroom, rich in lace and wool mats, containing a bedstead as glaring in brass as a fire-engine, a mirror draped with muslin and pink bows, and enough silver articles on the dressing-table to start a shop. After a discussion of the case with the doctor in a drawing-room which smelt like an empty church, I rushed off, leaving the doctor to detail the treatment we had advised, for I found – to my dismay – that I was twenty minutes late.

The second case was that of an exacting duke whom I had to visit at regular periods and, according to the ducal pleasure, I should be at the door at least one minute before the appointed hour struck. I was now hopelessly late and consequently flurried. On reaching the ducal abode I flew upstairs prepared to meet the storm. His Grace ignored my apologies and suggested, with uncouth irony, that I had been at a cricket match. He added that it was evident that I took no interest in him, that his sufferings were nothing to me, and concluded by asserting that if he had been dying I should not have hurried. I always regard remarks of this type as a symptom of disease rather than as a considered criticism of conduct, and therefore had little difficulty in bringing the duke to a less contentious frame of mind by reverting to that topic of the day – his engrossing disorder.

The duke never allowed his comfort to be in any way disturbed. He considered his disease as a personal affront to himself, and I therefore discussed it from the point of view of an unprovoked and indecent outrage. This he found very pleasing, although I failed to answer his repeated inquiry as to why His Grace the Duke of X should be afflicted in this rude and offensive manner. It was evident that his position should have exempted him from what was quite a vulgar disorder, and it was incomprehensible that he, of all people, should have been selected for this insult.

The interview over, I made my report to the duchess, who was in a little room adjacent to the hall. She followed me out to ask a final question just as I was on the point of taking my hat. The hat handed to me by the butler was, however, a new hat I had never seen before. It was of a shape I disliked. The butler, with due submission, said it was the hat I came in. I replied it was impossible, and, putting it on my head, showed that it was so small as to be absurd. The duchess, who was a lady of prompt convictions, exclaimed, 'Ridiculous; that was never your hat!' The butler could say no more: he was convicted of error. The duchess then seized upon the only other hat on the table and held it at arm's length. 'Whose is this?' she cried. 'Heavens, it is the shabbiest hat I ever saw! It cannot be yours.' (It was not.) Looking inside, she added, 'What a filthy hat! It is enough to poison the house.' Handing it to the butler as if it had been an infected rag, she exclaimed, 'Take it away and burn it!'

The butler did not at once convey this garbage to the flames, but remarked – as if talking in his sleep – 'There is a pianoforte tuner in the drawing-room.' The duchess stared with amazement at this inconsequent remark. Whereupon the buter added that the new hat I had rejected might possibly be his. He was at once sent up to confront the artist, whose aimless tinkling could be heard in the hall, with the further message that if the dirty hat should happen to be his he was never to enter the house again. The butler returned to say that the musician did not 'use' a hat. He wore a cap, which same he had produced from his pocket.

While the butler was away a great light had illumined the mind of the duchess. It appeared that Lord Andrew, her son-in-law, had called that afternoon with his wife. He had just left, his wife remaining behind. It was soon evident that the duchess had a grievance against her son-in-law. When the light fell upon her she exclaimed to me, 'I see it all now. This horrible hat is Andrew's. He has taken yours by mistake and has left this disgusting thing behind. It is just like him. He is the worst-dressed man in London, and this hat is just the kind he would wear.'

At this moment the daughter appeared. She had overheard her mother's decided views, and was proportionately indignant. She disdained to even look at the hat, preferring to deal with the indictment of Andrew on general grounds. She defended her husband from the charge of being unclean with no little show of temper. Without referring to the specific hat, she said she was positive, on a priori grounds, that Andrew would never wear a dirty hat. Her mother had no right to say such things. It was unjust and unkind.

The duchess was now fully roused. She was still more positive. This, she affirmed, was just the sort of thing Andrew would do – leave an old hat behind and take a good one. She would send him at once a note by a footman demanding the immediate return of my hat and the removal of his own offensive headgear.

The daughter, deeply hurt, had withdrawn from the discussion. I suggested that as Lady Andrew was about to go home she might inquire if a mistake had been made. Her Grace, however, was far too moved to listen to such moderation. She wanted to tell Andrew what she thought of him, and it was evident she had long been seeking the opportunity. So she at once stamped off to write the note. In the meanwhile I waited, gazing in great melancholy of mind at the two hats. The silent butler also kept his eyes fixed upon them with a gloom even deeper than mine. I had hinted that the new hat might belong to Lord Andrew, but the duchess had already disposed of that suggestion by remarking with assurance that Andrew never wore a new hat. The note was produced and at once dispatched by a footman.

I have no idea of the wording of the note, but I was satisfied that the duchess had not been ambiguous, and that she had told her son-in-law precisely what were her present views of him in a wider sense than could be expressed in terms of hats. The writing of the letter had relieved her. She was almost calm.

She now told the silent butler to fetch one of the duke's hats, so that I might have at least some decent covering to my bare head thus unscrupulously stripped by the unclean Andrew. The butler returned with a very smart hat of the duke's. It had apparently never been worn. It fitted me to perfection. In this vicarious coronet I regained my carriage. I felt almost kindly towards the duke now that I was wearing his best hat.

Next day I placed the ducal hat in a befitting hat-box and, having put on another hat of my own, was starting for the scene of the downfall of Lord Andrew. At my door a note was handed me. It was from the suburban doctor. He very courteously pointed out that I had taken his hat by mistake, and said he would be glad if I would return it at my convenience, as he had no other, and my hat came down over his eyes. It was a dreadful picture, that of a respected practitioner going his rounds with a hat resting on the bridge of his nose; but at least it cleared up the mystery of the new hat. The butler was right. In my anxiety at being late on the previous afternoon I was evidently not conscious that I was wearing a hat which must have looked like a thimble on the top of an egg.

On reaching the ducal residence I was received by the butler. He said nothing; but it seemed to me that he smiled immoderately for a butler. The two hats, the new and the dirty, were still on the table, but the duchess made no appearance. I returned the duke's hat with appropriate thanks and expressed regret for the stupid mistake I had made on the occasion of my last visit. I then placed the doctor's new hat I had repudiated in the hat-box ready for removal.

The full mystery was still unsolved, while the butler stood in the hall like a hypnotized sphinx. I said, in a light and casual way, 'And what about Lord Andrew? Did his lordship answer the note?' The butler replied, with extreme emphasis, 'He did indeed!' Poor duchess, I thought, what a pity she had been so violent and so hasty.

Still the dirty hat remained shrouded in mystery, so, pointing to it, I said to the butler, 'By the way, whose hat *is* that?' 'That hat, sir,' he replied, adopting the manner of a showman in a museum, 'that hat is the duke's. It is the hat His Grace always wears when he goes out in the morning.' 'But then,' I asked, 'why did you not tell the duchess so yesterday?' He replied, 'What, sir! After Her Grace had said that the hat was enough to poison the house! Not me!'

GENERAL NON-FICTION

	Godfrey Baseley	
0352303018	A COUNTRY COMPENDIUM	£1.50
	Linda Blandford	
0352301392	OIL SHEIKHS	95p
	Anthony Cave Brown	
0352396121	BODYGUARD OF LIES (Large Format)	£2.50*
Δ 0352302925	CLOSE ENCOUNTERS OF THE THIRD KIND	95p*
	Rodney Dale and Joan Gray	
035230345X	EDWARDIAN INVENTIONS	£2.95
	John Dean	
0352301368	BLIND AMBITION	£1.50*
	Dr Fitzhugh Dodson	
0352300124	HOW TO PARENT	75p*
	Trevor Donald	
0426190009	CONFESSIONS OF IDI AMIN	95p†
	L. Grant	
0427004349	THE BASIC BABY BOOK	95p
	H. R. Haldeman	
0352303247	THE ENDS OF POWER	£1.25*
	Paul Hammond and Patrick Hughes	
0352302674	UPON THE PUN (illus)	£1.25
	Clive Harold	
0352303506	THE UNINVITED	95p
	Xaviera Hollander	
0426168623	THE HAPPY HOOKER	80p*
0426163443	LETTERS TO THE HAPPY HOOKER	80p*
0426166787	XAVIERA ON THE BEST PART OF A MAN	80p*
0426134265	XAVIERA!	80p*
	Anne Fletcher	
0352303891	THE HAPPY HOOKER GOES TO WASHINGTON (F)	90p*
	Francis Huxley	
0352305010	THE WAY OF THE SACRED	£2.50*
	Paul Scanlon and Michael Gross	
Δ 0352304227	THE BOOK OF ALIEN	£1.95*
	Sharon Lawrence	
0352301627	SO YOU WANT TO BE A ROCK & ROLL STAR	95p*
	David Lewis	
0426087232	SEXPIONAGE	70p
0426087151	THE SECRET LIFE OF ADOLF HITLER	75p

† For sale in Britain and Ireland only.
* Not for sale in Canada. ● Reissues.
Δ Film & T.V. tie-ins.

Wyndham Books are obtainable from many booksellers and newsagents. If you have any difficulty please send purchase price plus postage on the scale below to:

Wyndham Cash Sales
P.O. Box 11
Falmouth
Cornwall
OR
Star Book Service
G.P.O. Box 29
Douglas
Isle of Man
British Isles

While every effort is made to keep prices low, it is sometimes necessary to increase prices at short notice. Wyndham Books reserve the right to show new retail prices on covers which may differ from those advertised in the text or elsewhere.

Postage and Packing Rate

UK: 30p for the first book, plus 15p per copy for each additional book ordered to a maximum charge of £1.29.
BFPO and Eire: 30p for the first book, plus 15p per copy for the next 6 books and thereafter 6p per book. **Overseas:** 50p for the first book and 15p per copy for each additional book.

These charges are subject to Post Office charge fluctuations.